THE INTELLIGENT PATIENT'S GUIDE TO THE DOCTOR–PATIENT RELATIONSHIP

Learning How to Talk
So Your Doctor Will Listen

BARBARA M. KORSCH, M.D. & CAROLINE HARDING

NEW YORK   OXFORD
OXFORD UNIVERSITY PRESS
1997

Oxford University Press

Oxford   New York
Athens   Auckland   Bangkok   Bogotá   Bombay
Buenos Aires   Calcutta   Cape Town   Dar es Salaam
Delhi   Florence   Hong Kong   Istanbul   Karachi
Kuala Lumpur   Madras   Madrid   Melbourne
Mexico City   Nairobi   Paris   Singapore
Taipei   Tokyo   Toronto   Warsaw

and associated companies in
Berlin   Ibadan

Published by Oxford University Press, Inc.
198 Madison Avenue, New York, New York 10016

Oxford is a registered trademark of Oxford University Press

Library of Congress Cataloging-in-Publication Data
Korsch, Barbara M.
The intelligent patient's guide to the doctor–patient relationship:
learning how to talk so your doctor will listen/
Barbara M. Korsch and Caroline Harding.
p.   cm.   Includes bibliographical references and index.
ISBN 0-19-510264-9
1. Physician and patient.   2. Consumer education.
3. Interpersonal communication.
I. Harding, Caroline.   II. Title.
R727.3.K67   1997   610.69'6—dc21   97-373

3 5 7 9 8 6 4 2

Printed in the United States of America
on acid-free paper

CONTENTS

▼
▼

ACKNOWLEDGMENTS

This book is based on fifty years of experience in medicine. Patients, their families, colleagues, and friends have all been my teachers. A large amount of what I know and what I experience comes from reading—science, but also important world literature, including fiction. It is not possible for me to trace the sources and influences that have actually shaped my own thinking.

Giving credit to selected individuals who have been significant in my professional life would mean omitting others who have been equally influential. But I wish to pay homage to the late Loren Stephens, a wise and sensitive teacher who inspired my interest and understanding of what "doctoring" is all about and who is responsible for many of the ideas in this book.

My colleagues at the Bayer Institute for Health Communication, especially Greg Carroll and Vaughn Keller, have been an invaluable resource.

I owe the reader an explanation regarding the case illustrations used in this work. The long dialogues come from literal transcripts of recorded medical visits. Shorter quotes are gleaned from medical practice, mostly my own, and sometimes that of colleagues as well as from the files of the Bayer Institute for Health Communication.

We have had to review a great many publications and wish to thank Doreen Keough, Health Sciences Librarian at Childrens Hospital Los Angeles. There has been no reference, no matter how old or how obscure, that she was not able to produce quickly.

There have been thousands of publications on the doctor–patient relationship since the 1940s. We will not attempt to review the literature, and cite original sources only in relation to specific research projects. For the interested reader we have suggested a few from the many excellent books that deal with the doctor–patient relationship in general. (See the Selected Readings at the end of the book.)

Most of all, we owe special gratitude to our editor, Joan Bossert. She has been a valuable collaborator throughout the preparation of this manu-script. Her support, contributions, and constructive criticisms have been invaluable. To our families and friends, especially Robert Ward III and Harding B. Michel, Ph.D., we are grateful for their having encouraged and sustained us during this work.

December 1996   B. K.
Los Angeles, California   C. H.

THE INTELLIGENT
PATIENT'S GUIDE TO
THE DOCTOR–PATIENT
RELATIONSHIP

POINT COUNTERPOINT

Listening to Both Sides

▼
▼

Why do we complain about our doctors? Why do they complain about us? What makes the doctor–patient relationship so complex? Well, for one thing, the doctor has more power than the patient, the doctor has more knowledge about the particular subject at hand than the patient, the patient is understandably anxious, the doctor has more responsibility, the doctor is prepared for the encounter, the patient is not, the doctor knows the ground rules, the patient does not. This book will increase your understanding of the relationship and the unwritten rules which dominate it.

But the medical setting itself creates many basic barriers to open, effective, and mutually satisfying communication. In addition, many small misunderstandings contribute to dissatisfaction on both sides, waste time, and ultimately adversely effect outcomes. Each individual in the interaction has perceptions of the other's behavior and very often the twain don't meet.

To see ourselves as others see us can help us to gain insight into what's going on and aid in our thinking about how to fix it. The same situation looks different to each side of the equation:

DOCTORS COMPLAIN	PATIENTS COMPLAIN
My patient rambles	*The doctor doesn't listen . . . .*
My patient doesn't do what I say.	*My doctor doesn't understand why I can't follow those instructions.*
She always has one more thing to talk about just as I'm about to walk out the door.	*If I remember something important, aren't I supposed to mention it?*
Will he ever get to the point?	*My doctor interrupts.*
My patient complains about things I can't control.	*He should be able to do something about the parking!*
There is no way of telling how much time I will have to spend with each patient.	*I had to wait so long, I feel like sending my doctor a bill.*
My patient blames me when she doesn't get better.	*I've had three appointments now, and I still feel terrible.*
My patient feels entitled and doesn't appreciate what I do for her.	*He gets paid to do it! He's not doing me any favors.*
My patient keeps relevant information from me.	*I'm not supposed to tell him! He's supposed to tell me!*
My patient expects me to make her husband stop drinking.	*I simply asked her to speak to Ted about his drinking.*
She comes on to me.	*I can't see why we can't be friends.*

DOCTORS COMPLAIN	PATIENTS COMPLAIN
Why do patients make appointments at the last minute and then complain about waiting?	*I can never get an appointment when I really need to see my doctor.*
The patient I'm seeing doesn't appreciate it if I interrupt to take a call.	*I really needed to talk to her and the nurse wouldn't put me through.*
I use humor to lighten things up.	*Sometimes I feel like my doctor is making fun of me.*
I always call my patients by their first names.	*I call him "Dr." Why don't I get the same respect?*
She's a doctor-shopper.	*I figure it's always best to get a second opinion. Two heads are better than one.*
I don't think he trusts me.	*Why should I trust him? I've only seen him twice. And for less than ten minutes each time.*
I have to concentrate on what I'm doing.	*I couldn't tell you what color his eyes are because he never looks at me.*
I give such careful and detailed explanations and he still doesn't understand.	*If only she'd speak English. She uses so many technical terms.*
Doing the physical and keeping accurate records take up my time.	*My doctor is the strong silent type.*
I make an effort to tell her what she did wrong so that she'll know better next time.	*He yells at me and makes me feel bad.*

DOCTORS COMPLAIN	PATIENTS COMPLAIN
Medicine is serious business.	*My doctor never smiles.*
I can't become emotional with every patient.	*He doesn't seem to care.*
I don't even have time to sit down.	*I wish the doctor would sit down when I'm talking to her.*
Every time this patient visits, there are a million questions that don't have anything to do with the visit.	*My doctor doesn't leave me any time for questions.*
That patient asks me the same question over and over.	*I never really get the answer I was hoping for.*
My office is on a tight schedule. I can't be sitting around waiting while they're getting undressed.	*He leaves me sitting there without my clothes on for too long!*
I don't have time for social chitchat.	*My doctor doesn't see me as a person.*
You can't expect me to remember every detail about each patient.	*My doctor forgets what I tell him.*
Sometimes I have to ask personal questions.	*My doctor embarrasses me.*
When it's something serious, I have to tell the patient what to do.	*My doctor makes decisions for me.*
There are no simple answers to most questions.	*He always hedges and never commits himself.*

DOCTORS COMPLAIN	PATIENTS COMPLAIN
I like educated patients, but I haven't got enough time to listen to everything they've heard somewhere.	*My doctor gets annoyed when I try to tell her what I know.*
When my patients have symptoms due to life stresses, instead of giving them medicine they don't need I try to help them understand.	*My doctor said it was all in my head.*
I have only so much time set aside for the visit and I try to concentrate on the patient's major concern.	*My doctor is always in such a hurry.*
I worry when patients self-medicate and don't really understand what they're doing.	*My doctor gets angry when I buy over-the-counter remedies.*
Unless I know that there is a medical reason for patients to stay home, I cannot sign excuses.	*My doctor refused to sign a paper saying I couldn't go to work.*
Ethically and legally, I cannot sign prescriptions when I haven't examined the patient recently.	*My doctor will not refill my prescription over the phone.*
It's unrealistic to expect doctors to actually like all of their patients.	*My doctor doesn't like me.*
Patients who come across as "poor little me" turn me off.	*When I'm sick, I do feel sorry for myself. Don't most people?*

DOCTORS COMPLAIN	PATIENTS COMPLAIN
I expect my patients to have a minimum of good sense.	*My doctor makes me feel stupid.*
I can't start the visit by telling my patient I only have fifteen minutes.	*My doctor never lets me know how much time she has. Then, without warning, time is up.*

DOCTORS MINIMIZE	PATIENTS EXAGGERATE
We have to do a few tests.	*"A few tests" means a whole day of painful procedures for me.*
The nurse will call you if there's anything to worry about.	*I found myself sitting by the phone wondering if they had forgotten.*
You may find it a little uncomfortable.	*I was in complete agony.*
You may have to wait a little while.	*Be prepared for 2½ hours.*
The doctor will be here in a minute.	*A half hour later, you are still waiting.*
The doctor says, "Oh, I don't think you'll need any Novocaine while I sew up this little cut."	*The next thing you know, you are hurting but too embarrassed to say anything.*
The doctor says, "We don't need to put you in the hospital for this procedure. It's not serious."	*I could hardly make it home.*
This medicine may make you drowsy.	*I barely could see straight!*

Managed Care

Not only do doctors and patients have complaints in relation to one another, but they also have different perceptions of the rapidly changing health-care system.

DOCTORS COMPLAIN	PATIENTS COMPLAIN
I have no control over which patients come to my practice.	*I can't even choose my own doctor anymore.*
I'm not always free to refer patients for the tests and consultations they request.	*My doctor refused to send me to a specialist.*
I'm given too little time per patient. The way they set up the office is really not to my taste, but I have to fit in.	*He never has enough time. I don't like his new office. It's too busy and too impersonal.*
I miss having my own nurse and receptionist.	*I don't know anyone who works in my doctor's office anymore.*
They drive me crazy with all the things I have to fill out—all the forms and paperwork!	*It's ridiculous! When I get there all I do is fill out forms.*
The way they schedule patients, it's hard to develop a good relationship.	*I don't really even know my doctor anymore.*
I'm booked so heavily that I can't even save any openings for my own patients.	*If I need to see my doctor on short notice, forget it.*
Just when I get a good working relationship going with a patient, he or she changes jobs and can't come back.	*In my new job, I can't go to my own doctor anymore.*

DOCTORS COMPLAIN	PATIENTS COMPLAIN
Patients wait so long they are angry before they come to see me.	*They make me wait so long, I wonder why I bother getting there on time.*
When the personnel is rude to a patient they take it out on me.	*I think the doctor should be able to control how his nurse treats me.*

So, is there something wrong with you or is it your doctor? What makes doctors act the way they do? What makes you act the way you do? You're anxious. The doctor's rushed. You both react differently for a variety of reasons: time pressures, anxiety about being sick, the doctor's sense of responsibility for his or her patients where there is no room for mistakes. The situation, the power imbalance, the emotions that go into it, and practical details all conspire to make both doctor and patient feel on edge.

Under ordinary circumstances, doctors and patients are each doing their best to live up to their responsibility. But besides the basic inequities in power, medical knowledge, feelings about the medical visit, who is paying whom, who chose whom, there are a lot of unnecessary smaller barriers to communication that can be avoided by greater understanding, trying harder, increased sensitivity, and more imagination.

Certainly, there are general rules that prevail in medical practice, but there are no set rules for the individual encounter between patient and physician. This book is about realizing what goes on between you and your physician—inside you, inside your doctor, and inside the medical setting. A better understanding of all these things should liberate you to make the best possible use of your opportunities when you see your doctor.

SO, WHAT DID THE
DOCTOR SAY?

Have you ever walked out of the doctor's office and realized that you didn't really know what happened? Many of us have experienced visits when, from the moment the doctor enters the room, nothing seems to go as we had planned. Why is it that we often leave the doctor's office feeling that we didn't have the opportunity to ask all the questions we had been thinking about before the appointment? How many times have you almost been home before realizing,

"Oh no, I forgot to ask about . . ."?

Or, after a doctor's appointment, you find yourself at a loss for words when someone asks,

"So, what did the doctor say?"

Perhaps you left without having the chance to explain why you really wanted to see him or her in the first place.

In most Western countries, we have access to highly trained and competent doctors. Why is it, then, that we hardly ever meet anyone with something to say that's positive? Did you know that more lawsuits today can be traced to communication difficulties between doctors and patients than technical medical errors? This chapter will raise many questions about our experiences with doctors, introduce some of the critical issues in the doctor–patient relationship, and shed light on some of the most common misunderstandings we have with doctors. Why is it that we sometimes have difficulty communicating with our doctors—and why do they have trouble communicating with us?

As both a physician and a professor of medicine, I interview a lot of young doctors and one of the questions I always ask is,

"Why did you want to be a doctor?"

The most common answer is,

"I like science and I like people."

That's exactly the answer I gave more than fifty years ago when I was entering medical school. Like everyone else, I thought that the science was all in the chemistry, the anatomy, the physiology, and the pathology. But what I have discovered over the years is that science is also about people. And if you are truly interested in helping your patients, it takes science, a very sophisticated science, to understand them as *people.*

Most doctors are excellent technicians, adept at diagnosing and treating illnesses and performing complex procedures. Just think of the skill and precision required for modern eye surgery, a quadruple cardiac bypass, or the painstaking reattachment of a severed digit. Unfortunately, many of those very talented and dexterous doctors are not as adept when it comes to communicating with their patients.

While the main responsibility for effective communication lies with physicians, all of us need to remember that communication is a two-way street. Patients have to hold up their end. When communication breaks down between a doctor and patient, it's not always because of poor skills on the part of the physician. There are problems that arise during an encounter for which both doctor and patient are responsible. As patients, we do have a great many opportunities to take an active role in improving the communication process.

Discovering the Problem

I have spent most of my professional life studying interactions between doctors and patients. My interest began in the early 1950s when I headed a large outpatient department at Cornell University New York Hospital Medical Center. As I reviewed patient charts at the end of each day, I was astonished by what I found. After waiting to see their doctors, answering a great many questions, going through long physical examinations, suffering through the inevitable lab tests, making their next appointments, and paying for their visits, many patients were ignoring their doctor's advice and often not even coming back.

What percentage of patients were not complying? In those early days, the field of doctor–patient communication had not even begun to develop. I was just discovering the phenomenon and was not yet taking a formal count of noncompliant patients. But in the coming years, as I looked further into the problem, I put together a large research team and we began to count and measure. Other investigators also became interested. Numerous studies have demonstrated that between one-third and two-thirds of patients in most clinical situations were not satisfied and did not follow through on medical advice. In my initial investigation, my primary interest was to understand the phenomenon and find out what was going wrong. What was it about the doctor or the patient that caused these communication breakdowns?

At first, we could not fathom where the problem lay. Obviously, something we were doing wasn't working. The physicians had all taken complete medical histories, performed meticulous physical examinations, and given correct medical advice. Yet the patients weren't benefiting from our expert services. I was frequently called down to the emergency room and even there, where some of the children were desperately ill, our patients' parents were at times unwilling to accept our advice. Here were children with potentially life-threatening illnesses and their parents were taking them home rather than allowing them to be admitted to the hospital! I remember the listless toddler with sunken eyes suspected of having meningitis. When we began urgently preparing him for a spinal tap, his mother refused to sign permission and took him home. And the child with persistent abdominal pain that we suspected was being caused by an abscessed appendix. Her parents signed her out "against medical advice," a phrase we wrote so often that we used the abbreviation AMA. Had we failed to convince these parents that their children's lives were in danger? What were their reasons for not cooperating? And why weren't our other scheduled patients coming back?

It didn't satisfy me to label these patients uncooperative, which was the traditional explanation. Instead, I decided to begin looking in detail at the actual interaction between physicians and their patients. I developed a series of questions for the patients so that they could comment about their doctors and the care they had received. The patients we first approached were hesitant to answer my questions because they were afraid their criticisms would get back to the doctors. Not only were they apprehensive that their doctors might be offended, they actually worried that their treatment might suffer. When we reassured them that the interviews were strictly confidential, they began discussing their experiences with medical visits more openly. I started by asking questions that would elicit positive responses:

> "What were some of the things you liked about your visit with the doctor today? Did your doctor understand how concerned you were?"

And then I eased into the touchy areas:

> "What were some of the things you didn't like? Do you think you will be able to do what the doctor asked you to do? Would you come back to see this particular doctor?"

Although there were quite a few patients with good things to say about their doctors, they were outnumbered by those who had criticisms, especially relating to their doctors' lack of interpersonal skills:

> "He seemed to be in such a hurry . . . and he kept interrupting me."

"How could I know whether the doctor understood how concerned I was because all she did was blame me!"
"He said I needed to follow the treatment every three hours, but he didn't seem to listen when I said I couldn't do it at work."

Sound familiar? The problems patients were having with their doctors almost fifty years ago are not much different from those we have today with our own doctors. People have the tendency to look back fondly at "the old-fashioned doc"—the friendly, white-haired, small-town doctor with the gentle bedside manner who carried his black bag through television programs and movies half a century ago. Some people believe that he was the perfect communicator. But did he ever really exist?

Quite a few of us will stand up and enthusiastically defend our own doctors; we develop loyalties to them, especially the ones we know the best: our primary care doctors, family doctors, sometimes even such specialists as obstetricians. By the same token, doctors also become extremely loyal to their patients. The young doctors in the clinic refer to their own patients as "my patient" and get very upset if there is a system problem that causes "their" patient to be kept waiting for an hour in registration, or when they find out that "their" patient tried to call and was unable to get through. So, despite all the communication breakdowns and specific causes for dissatisfaction, there is also loyalty on both sides of the relationship.

One of the consistent sources for dissatisfaction in patients has been the discrepancy between their expectations and those of their physicians. Over the years, my rapidly growing research team and I made thousands of audio and videotapes of actual interactions between patients and doctors; we have also interviewed them individually at length. What we found was that they each have very different expectations. Doctors may focus exclusively on the patients' overt physical health problems and leave patients feeling that their underlying concerns and anxieties have been ignored. Technology and the biological, scientific basis of medicine have developed so fast and so dramatically that they are now what drives medical practice at the expense of many physicians' understanding of their patients. And when a physician does not have a thorough understanding of a patient's problem, it becomes difficult to form an effective working relationship.

The Current Scene

Most of us could come up with a number of heartfelt complaints about our doctors. No matter where I am—parties, airports, even grocery stores—if word gets out that I study doctor–patient communication problems, I am pursued by the many people who are convinced that they have *the* most dramatic story to tell. In a matter of moments, a reception I attended recently turned into a doctor-bashing free-for-all:

> *"You wouldn't believe what the internist said to me yesterday . . . ."*
> *"He doesn't treat me like a human being with feelings."*
> *"She didn't seem to listen to a word I said."*
> *"The gynecologist made me feel so stupid. . . . I wish he would act as if he cared about me."*
> *"Here I waited and waited to see the doctor and, when I finally got in, she didn't answer any of my questions."*
> *"I went to find out what's the matter with me, then I couldn't understand what he was talking about."*

Strangers come up to me and complain about their doctors. Just as I was about to board a plane for England not long ago, a young doctor who was traveling with me told the airline reservation agent that I was on my way to give a seminar about doctor–patient communication. The reservation agent immediately stopped work on my ticket and said, *"Have I got a good one for you!"*

My heart sank. I was about to hear another tale of woe. She launched into a story about having finally selected a woman gynecologist because her male doctor had never shown any empathy or concern about her condition. Her expectations were unfortunately dashed. Not only was her new female doctor abrupt, she didn't seem to listen to her problems, and she even told her that her menopausal symptoms were *"all in your head."* The poor agent had been greatly disappointed to find that her new female doctor was worse than the man had ever been.

Most people don't realize that even doctors are not immune to being treated badly by their own doctors. When I developed glaucoma after having eye surgery, my doctor was less than sympathetic. When he saw how upset I was, he quipped, *"What do you expect; nothing's ever simple when doctors get sick. That's why I hate to take care of doctors."*

Before one of my appointments, I had prepared a list of questions for the doctor about my condition. Because my mother had gone blind in the last ten years of her life, I was naturally very concerned. But when I got into his office and pulled out my list, he abruptly cut me off with, *"Oh no. Are we going to have to play twenty questions again?"*

You can imagine how, after that scathing comment, I walked out of his office, my questions unanswered, extremely frustrated and angry. Although this doctor was an expert technician and surgeon, my faith in his general competence had diminished. I felt so brutalized that I never wanted to see him again. My respect for him was gone and I knew that if he had understood anything about my feelings, he could never have spoken to me the way he did.

Why is it that doctors sometimes seem so unresponsive? Is it impatience or lack of concern? I've heard many patients complain that when they began talking about something that was really bothering them, the doctor cut them off with,

"Don't worry, it's nothing serious."

The doctor means to be reassuring, but reassurance can sound hollow when you feel that the doctor did not really understand. There are other times when the doctor seems to be busy reading your chart and making notes while you are trying to explain something. How could he possibly be listening?

Many of the young doctors I taught have not thought of the role of the physician as one of being a listener; as a result, they have come across as nonresponsive to patients. They are eager to give patients good advice and lectures about health behavior:

"You really must get your cholesterol down . . . try to find time to get more exercise . . . cut down on red meat . . . do I need to explain what you're doing to yourself by your continued smoking?"

It takes courage and persistence to get doctors to listen to our health concerns and anxieties. Doctors want to get right to the point—*"How high was the fever? When did you first notice it?"*

They're trained to focus on the medical task at hand and patients may interpret their seemingly detached behavior to mean, *Anything else you want to talk about is none of my business.* So while patients feel that some important issues have not been addressed because the doctor seemed uninterested, in fact doctors need to focus their attention on the medical task. As patients, we do have the right to decide what we want the doctor to hear. What we have to say is important and we feel that the doctor should pay attention! On the other hand, doctors must be able to get the information they require because they have a limited amount of time in which to take care of us.

While doctors are not responsible for dealing with separate family problems or unrelated emotional problems, they do have to take into account who their patients are, as well as the resources and limitations involved in their life situations. They need to be able to individualize a patient's treatment plan.

In many situations, whether we are taking classes or bringing our cars to auto mechanics, it helps to have the people we interact with understand who we are and why we are there. When you take your car in for service, for example, you feel the need to explain why you need it back as quickly as possible:

> *"I'll be late for my job."*
> *"I'm scheduled for an important meeting."*
> *"I'm supposed to pick someone up from the airport."*

Doctor–patient encounters rarely involve only the immediate task at hand, even in very task-oriented visits. If a child, for instance, is taken to the emergency room with a leg laceration and the doctor simply injects Novocaine and sews up the cut without attempting to find out anything other than what she needs to know medically, she may miss out on valuable information. Perhaps the parents could have provided details about how the accident happened that would have been useful to the physician in counseling them about how to prevent future accidents.

In a different setting, when a doctor asks a patient a few questions about her background, and she launches into a long saga about her troubled childhood, the physician has no other choice but to interrupt, feeling inundated with too much information. The patient then feels put off. Each situation will be different—doctors will have varying amounts of time to spend with patients, and patients will have different issues they feel they need to communicate.

What is appropriate for one encounter is frequently not appropriate for another. It depends on the setting and the purpose of the visit—one patient is extremely ill and needs hospitalization, the next has simply come in for a routine checkup, and another is in for her follow-up after last week's surgery. The doctor certainly knows what he needs to explore, but the patient also knows what he wants to get across. Quite often, a patient will volunteer essential information that the doctor had not expected or asked for, something that turns out to be important to future health care. And if the physician comes across as impersonal and uncaring, that attitude will not be as likely to promote the patient's motivation and cooperation in obtaining the follow-up care needed.

When Doctors Don't Respond to Concerns

Faced with patients who express strong emotions, doctors may become uncomfortable and often do what a teacher of mine called "escape into chronology" or "escape into technology."[1] They zero in on the time sequence of particular symptoms or focus on some technical aspect of the illness, such as the number of degrees of temperature elevation or details of medication dosage. An upset woman explained to her internist:

> *"Oh, when it happened, I was so depressed I thought I might kill myself. My husband had left and I was all alone and my child was sick."*

Escaping into chronology, the doctor promptly changed the subject with,

> *"Was that the year you moved from Texas?"*

A mother visiting a pediatrician was queried,

DOCTOR: *You have another son who came here?*

MOTHER: *Yes, my son came here.*

DOCTOR: *Is your son still coming here for care?*

MOTHER: *No, my son is deceased.*

DOCTOR: *What happened to your son?*

MOTHER: *He was shot in the head.*

Seemingly unresponsive to what he had just been told, the doctor continued calmly:

DOCTOR: *Now, this is how I want you to give the baby vitamins. Fill the little dropper up to where it is marked 0.6 cc and then . . . .*

As you can see, after learning that his patient's brother had recently been killed, the doctor promptly went on to deliver careful instruction to the mother about how to give vitamins to her baby. Why didn't this experienced doctor offer any comforting words or at least say he was sorry? Is it because he did not care about the mother's loss? Perhaps he had fallen behind in his schedule? Or maybe he did not feel comfortable discussing the child's death? Unfortunately, he most likely never learned the skills necessary for responding to human tragedy. He not only cut himself off from offering the appropriate reassurance, but also from inquiring about the nature of the accident and its implication for the future safety of his patient and the family.

Doctors do a lot more talking than listening. They see themselves as educators and as task-oriented doers, trained to help patients by doing things for them. "Find it and fix it" is their motto. In medical circles, the cardinal sin is to miss a diagnosis. If a doctor does not discover something that is physically wrong with a patient and someone else does, that doctor is subject to severe criticism. Consequently, many doctors concentrate primarily on finding out what's wrong. Their training does not encourage or develop the sensitivity needed to look at the patient as a person and realize how scared or how alone he or she may feel with their problem.

Taking the time to listen is difficult. For some doctors in certain settings—a high-pressure specialist's office, an HMO where the doctor's time is limited—it is next to impossible. But even in short patient visits, it is possible for a doctor with good listening skills to satisfy patients by being alert to their underlying concerns and responding to them.

In one of my cases, a mother tries to tell her doctor that her three-week-old baby is vomiting. She had been told that when newborn infants vomit, their stomachs may rupture. The mother wants to make the doctor understand that her baby has not been able to keep anything down for over twenty-four hours. Unaware of her distress and persistent pleas, the doctor asks her only technical questions relating to the danger of dehydration.

MOTHER: *Everything he takes in comes back up!*

DOCTOR: *Does he have a temperature?*

MOTHER: *Even water comes back up!*

DOCTOR: *Has he urinated today?*

MOTHER: *He threw up all night long!*

DOCTOR: *When he cries, are there tears?*

MOTHER: *What should I do if he keeps on throwing up?*

When we interviewed the mother after the appointment, she said, *"He never did understand that my baby was vomiting all the time!"* While the doctor did do a good technical job of finding out what was physically wrong, he neglected to address the mother's major concern and she felt he had failed to listen. And when patients feel a doctor does not know what their problems really are, why should they accept the doctor's solution?

In another case, a mother and father are told that their baby has a heart murmur. The young woman doctor gives a confusing explanation using many complex medical terms and offers neither comfort nor reassurance. She fails to listen and respond to their questions and concerns even though they are visibly frightened.

FATHER: *How does his heart sound?*

DOCTOR: *Sounds pretty good. He's got a little murmur there. I'm not sure what it is. It's . . . it, uh . . . could just be a little hole in his heart.*

MOTHER: *Is that very dangerous when you have a hole in your heart?*

DOCTOR: *No, because I think it's the upper chamber, and if it's the upper chamber, it means nothing.*

MOTHER: *Oh.*

DOCTOR: *Otherwise they just grow up and they repair them.*

MOTHER: *What would cause a hole in his heart?*

DOCTOR: *H'm?*

MOTHER: *What was it that caused the hole in his heart?*

DOCTOR: *It's 'cause . . . uh . . . just developmental, when they're uh . . . .*

MOTHER: *M-h'm.*

DOCTOR: *There's a little membrane that comes down, and if it's the upper chamber there's a membrane that comes down, one from each direction. And sometimes they don't quite meet, and so there's either a hole at the top or a hole at the bottom and then . . . it really . . . uh . . . almost never causes any trouble.*

MOTHER: *Oh.*

DOCTOR: *It's uh . . . one thing that they never get SBE from . . . it's only the heart lesion in which they don't.*

MOTHER: *Uh-huh.*

DOCTOR: *And uh . . . they grow up to be normal.*

MOTHER: *Oh, good.*

DOCTOR: *And uh . . . if anything happens, they can always catheterize them and make sure that's what it is, or do heart surgery.*

MOTHER: *Yeah.*

DOCTOR: *Really no problem with it. They almost never get into trouble so . . .*

MOTHER: *Do you think that he might have developed the murmur being that my husband and I both have a murmur?*

DOCTOR: *No.*

MOTHER: *No. Oh, it's not hereditary then?*

DOCTOR: *No.*

MOTHER: *Oh, I see.*

DOCTOR: *It is true that certain people . . . tendency to rheumatic fever, for instance.*

MOTHER: *Mmm.*

DOCTOR: *There is a tendency for the abnormal antigen-antibody reactions to be inherited, and therefore they can sometimes be more susceptible.*

MOTHER: *Oh, I see. That wouldn't mean anything if uh . . . I would . . . I'm Rh negative and he's positive. It wouldn't mean anything in that line, would it?*

DOCTOR: *Unh-unh.*

MOTHER: *No? Okay.*

DOCTOR: *No. The only thing you have to worry about is other babies.*

MOTHER: *M-h'm.*

DOCTOR: *Watch your Coombs and things.*

MOTHER: *Watch my what?*

DOCTOR: *Your titres . . . Coombs titres.*

MOTHER: *Oh, yeah.*

DOCTOR: *Have you ever had a blood transfusion?*

MOTHER: *No.*

DOCTOR: *Oh, you'll probably be all right, I think, for a while.*

MOTHER: *Oh.*

DOCTOR: *No . . . A heart murmur is by itself.*

MOTHER: *M-hm.*

DOCTOR: *It's just developmental.*

MOTHER: *Yeah.*

DOCTOR: *At first I thought it might be functional, the way you described it, but a functional murmur is heard down at the bottom of the heart and his is heard more up here at the top . . . .*

MOTHER: *Ohh.*

DOCTOR: *. . . and along the sides. So I think you can probably . . . but it's without a thrill so it means he probably . . .*

MOTHER: *M-hm.*

DOCTOR: *In fact, it may even close off at times.*

MOTHER: *Yeah?*

DOCTOR: *'Cause sometimes the pressure in their hearts aren't enough to make them open.*

MOTHER: *Mmm.*

DOCTOR: *And sometimes it's only with pressure and gradient differences. These things open and you can hear a murmur.*

MOTHER: *Oh. I see.*

DOCTOR: *So . . . a lot of murmurs are heard at birth that are buried at six weeks.*

MOTHER: *Yeah? Well! I didn't know that.*

DOCTOR: *Even some of your terminal . . . your blue babies sometimes don't turn blue 'til they're three or four weeks old.*

MOTHER: *Oh yeah?*

DOCTOR: *'Cause of pressure gradients.*

MOTHER: *M-hm. Oh my gosh.*

Doctor and patient are not speaking the same language. One is speaking "medical" while the other is speaking English. Any parent would have difficulty understanding this doctor. What do "SBE" and "Coombs titres" mean? Not knowing Latin and not having been medically trained, the patient is lost. And scared. How did the parents feel when the doctor made ominous references to other critically ill children using the words *terminal* and *blue babies?* And terms like catheterize, heart surgery, heart lesions, rheumatic fever, and abnormal antigen-antibody reactions are alarming.

Some doctors believe that patients should be frightened a little so that they will do what the doctor tells them. Could that be what this doctor intended? Or was she unaware of how frightened the parents were? The doctor did most of the talking, leaving little opportunity to ask questions. Although she attempted to explain the nature of the child's heart problem at length, she did not have the necessary communication skills to make the explanation helpful to the parents.

What could the parents have done to improve communication? Although there are many ways in which they could have changed the direction of the encounter, when patients are given frightening news about possible life-threatening illness in themselves or their children, they intuitively resist from coming across as too challenging or aggressive. They are afraid, they need the doctor, and they do not want to risk offending him or her. It is difficult for patients to judge when more challenging behavior will result in improved communication or when it will come across as threatening to the doctor and result in a new communication barrier. The more serious the health threat, the less likely a patient will take a chance on challenging the doctor. This mother did try valiantly to get answers to three of her questions. The first expressed her fears:

"Is that very dangerous when you have a hole in your heart?"

If the doctor had really been listening, she would have realized how anxious the mother was and offered reassurance. Instead, after an exchange in which the doctor first tells her that she does not think the child is in danger because she believes the hole is in the upper chamber, *"which means nothing,"* she then creates uncertainty by saying,

"Otherwise they just grow up and they repair them."

This is when the mother asks:

"What would cause a hole in his heart?"

Not receiving an answer, she asks again,

"What was it that caused the hole in his heart?"

I have observed that usually when a doctor or patient has to repeat some-thing more than two times, there has been a breakdown in communication. Or, if a doctor finds that he has to ask a question three times, it often means that the patient did not understand the first time. If a doctor gives the same advice three times and the patient does not make an appropriate response, there is something wrong with the way that doctor is communicating. In our case, the mother did ask the same question twice, but still did not get a satisfactory answer. The doctor began, *"It's 'cause . . . uh . . . just developmen-tal, when they're uh . . ."* and then again attempted to answer the question, this time with a confusing anatomical description of how membranes can create holes by not meeting properly.

As a patient, if you find that you have to raise an issue two or three times and still do not get through, you need to say to the doctor,

> *"I've been trying to tell you about this for the last few minutes and I really need for you to hear me right now."*

Or, if the doctor has already attended to the primary reasons for your visit and the question you're asking is one that can wait, it may help to tell your-self,

> *Maybe this is not the right time to talk about it, so I must make sure to remember my question for next time.*

To the mother of the baby with the heart murmur, the doctor gives complex and confusing explanations, permitting the mother only monosyllabic replies. Still, the mother does try to ask another question. She is worried that she and her husband are to blame:

> *"Do you think that he might have developed the murmur being that my husband and I both have a murmur?"*

The doctor answers with a curt, *"No,"* and proceeds to discuss rheumatic fever and abnormal antigen-antibody reactions. This prompts the mother to ask,

> *"That wouldn't mean anything if uh . . . I would . . . I'm Rh negative and he's positive. It wouldn't mean anything in that line, would it?"*

Even though the mother's questions were relevant, she failed to get a response and gave up. Without being too confrontational, she could have insisted,

> *"We've been in here quite a long time and you've told us a lot of important things but they were hard for us to understand. There are a couple of questions we really need answers to. Could you tell us what you think is wrong with our baby and what you think caused it?"*

This would have prompted the doctor to reassure the parents that their murmurs and blood type have nothing to do with their baby's problem and that they should not blame themselves. The mother might then have asked,

> *"Is there anything special we need to do?"*

Had this doctor been more in tune with her patients' feelings, she also would have spent a few minutes responding to their fears:

> *"Learning that there is something wrong with your baby's heart must be frightening for you. I wish that I could give you a definite diagnosis and more reassurance, but until we have done some tests and I have discussed this with a heart specialist, I don't have enough information to do that. . . . If you have any questions for me in the meantime, please call."*

At the end of the visit, this doctor should have taken a moment to acknowledge the amount of information she had given them, reassured them that their baby was doing fine, and made herself available to answer any further questions they might have had. Instead, this doctor ended the interview by mentioning blue babies and pressure gradients, leaving the parents even more anxious and confused:

"M-hm. Oh my gosh."

During the visit, the doctor hardly ever looked at the parents. She became immersed in the complexity of the medical problem. If she had just taken a few moments to glance at their facial expressions, she would have seen how anxious they were. Through the years, I have developed a skill that has been helpful to me both as a doctor and a patient. In educational terminology, we refer to it as *metacognition,* and it means simply that you are aware of what you are doing as you do it and are consciously planning your next move. When I am with a patient, as I talk I think about the result I am looking for, how far the interview has progressed, how I am speaking, and how the patient is listening and responding. If something goes wrong, I am then able to realize it quickly. If I observe the patient's facial expressions and body language changing, if I notice my own voice getting louder or realize that I'm beginning to feel frustrated, then I stop myself and begin thinking about how to get back on the right track.

Getting Your Story Across

Have *you* ever left the doctor's office without finding out what was the matter? You fill out the necessary forms, answer the doctor's questions, and go through an extensive physical examination. Then you are given a brief explanation, perhaps a prescription, and you are on your own. Later, when a friend or family member asks you what the doctor said, you hesitate and realize that you're not really sure. A good number of the patients I have interviewed felt they didn't really get a diagnosis:

"But, the doctor never did tell me what was the matter!"

Doctors use phrases that are meant to be diagnostic statements but don't mean much to patients because they're in a language they can't understand:

"I think this may just be viral . . . ." (This may just be a cold.)
"He probably has bronchitis or RAD." (It looks like asthma.)
"This kind of pain is usually only functional." (This pain is typically insignificant or psychosomatic.)

And often the doctor is in a hurry and the patient is either too embarrassed to ask for an explanation or is not given the opportunity to do so.

It has been demonstrated consistently that the opening of the medical visit, the first few minutes you spend with your doctor, are tremendously important. During those initial minutes, the kind of rapport you will have is established and the doctor sets the pace for the interview. Ideally, the doctor should devote the beginning of the visit to letting you tell your story. In reality, most doctors will not listen to your concerns very long before interrupting.

In one study conducted in an internal medicine practice, scientists found that physicians, on the average, listened to patients' concerns for about eighteen seconds.[2] I've asked doctors how long they think patients would talk if allowed to go uninterrupted. Their typical reply:

"They'll go on and on!"

Yet, the investigation demonstrated that, if allowed to go uninterrupted, patients will talk for an average of two and a half minutes. If you time yourself, you'll find that two and a half minutes is actually quite a long time and it gives you a chance to cover a lot. Although doctors feel that they do not have enough time to listen, it has been found that if the patient's story is elicited early in an open-ended, nonjudgmental, and facilitating way, the visit will actually take less time.

Depending on the doctor's style, the particular practice setting, the purpose of the visit, and how much time your physician has to spend, you will be given a certain amount of time in which to discuss your concerns. Doctors sometimes use a lot of "yes" and "no" questions that they hope will make for short, effective information gathering. For certain aspects of the medical history this is appropriate, but when it predominates, patients tend to feel they have been interrogated instead of interviewed. It's also not uncommon for patients to be faced with doctors who put words in their mouths because they think it will get them the specific facts they need faster. But what actually happens is that they cut out valuable information that the patient might have provided.

DOCTOR: *When you had that bellyache, where was it?*

PATIENT: *Well, it was . . . .*

DOCTOR: *Mostly around your umbilicus?*

PATIENT: *And then it spread to my . . .*

DOCTOR: *But you were not constipated?*

PATIENT: *No . . . .*

It would be better for the physician to open up the discussion by allowing you to voice your own questions and thoughts:

PATIENT: *I've had this awful stomachache.*

DOCTOR: *Can you tell me some more about that?*

PATIENT: *Well, it was a cramping pain that kept on for several hours . . . .*

If the doctor uses open-ended questions and facilitating replies, you are given the opportunity to begin telling your story. When doctors reflect their patients' feelings, it encourages them to continue:

PATIENT: *Oh, you just can't imagine how depressed I was when it happened.*

DOCTOR: *I can understand that you would be very depressed.*

PATIENT: *I finally recovered from the surgery and now this.*

What can you, as a patient, do when a physician puts words in your mouth or begins asking you "yes" or "no" questions? In the first few minutes, it is difficult to take the initiative to reprogram your doctor, for instance, by interrupting with,

"But if you'd just let me tell you . . . ."

The best approach is to be aware of what is going on and not let yourself be discouraged about telling your story. Then, whenever you can, say to your physician:

"It would make me feel better to tell you what it was really like, and besides, there were some other things I didn't have the chance to tell you about."

Many patients go to their appointments without having thought through what exactly it is that they expect help with:

"I'm feeling so sick. . . . What do I do? . . . I hope the doctor helps me."

Not only does this make it harder for you, it makes it more difficult for the doctor to assist you. Before going to your appointment, spend some time formulating your concerns, taking into consideration the most important points you want to get across. Give some thought to what you need help with. Perhaps even talk it over with someone. You may not have the opportunity to ask your doctor everything, so don't come up with too many questions. Concentrate instead on the most important ones that you want answered. In one research project,[3] patients given a few minutes with a physician's assistant who helped them focus on their most pertinent questions before the visit demonstrated that these patients usually had only two or three major questions.

It is also important to think about any questions you might hesitate to ask. Patients are often embarrassed to ask certain things. They may feel intimidated by their doctors or uncomfortable with the subject matter they want to raise. For instance, if you haven't been taking the medicine the doctor prescribed, you may hesitate to broach the subject. It is important for patients and doctors to realize that it is the doctor's job to understand, not to judge. If the doctor has not told you what to do if you forget to take your medicine, be sure to bring up that issue:

"What should I do if I forget to take my medicine? Should I double it up the next time?"

Patients also feel embarrassed about not having understood something the doctor has said. There are tactful ways, without blaming the doctor, of bringing this to his or her attention.

"You know, I asked you this last time and you did give me an answer, but when I thought about it, I realized that I really didn't understand."

Taking Steps to Improve the Relationship

Although the interactions you have with your doctor can be frustrating, this relationship is one of the most important ones you will ever have. Unfortunately, many people avoid doctors when they know they shouldn't, and others bypass doctors by going to chiropractors and herbalists. These alternative healers are offering something to patients that the medical profession may not have. They make the effort to communicate well with people who visit them as well as provide understanding and compassion. Of course, good communication is not always enough. We all want the best medical care available, but we may not get it when we are not happy with our doctors.

What has happened to the doctor–patient relationship? There are changes in the systems for health-care delivery that are definitely going to make it more difficult for people to have satisfying, long-term relationships with their doctors. Under managed health care, the relationship between patients and doctors is changing—we often are unable to choose our doctors, doctors are inundated with rules, regulations, and pressures, and, above all, our doctors have very little time with us.

In the face of all these stresses, making communication in the doctor–patient relationship as effective as possible is going to be more important than ever. As patients, are we to reach out more to understand our doctors? Shouldn't our doctors make more of an effort to understand and respond to us? With less time available and our health at stake, we need to learn more about our relationships with doctors, what to expect from them, why things go wrong, and what can be done to make it better. In fact, when all is said and done, it is not the actual health care that people complain about in this country. We have perhaps the best technical expertise available. What people complain about is the lack of communication and the psychological issues.

In many ways, doctors live in a world of their own with a different language, value system, goals, and ways of achieving results. When we go to them for help, we need to talk about our experiences with illness and express our feelings, anxieties, and concerns—and we rarely have enough opportunity to do so. Doctors have too little time and need to get down to business. We each have our own agendas and, unfortunately, they often conflict.

This book is not about the doctor or the patient. It's about what goes on between them and why we need to be aware of the common breakdowns in communication so that we can overcome them. It is important to remember that our relationships with doctors are not one-sided. When we are unhappy with them, they are usually not happy with us either. We each have difficult roles. For patients, it is frightening to be sick. We may have to place our trust in the hands of someone we don't know very well or may never have even met before. For doctors, they are challenged each and every time they walk into an examination room or stop at a hospital bed. They are in constant demand day and night to respond to their patients' needs. At the same time, they have to adapt to increasing pressures from the changing health-care system. And so do we.

The relationship between doctors and patients is powerful and complex. When you get right down to it, it's really a partnership. We depend on them and they depend on us. There are times in our lives when the relationship is absolutely crucial. It has the potential of making us healthier and helping us to live longer. And to realize that potential, we—and by "we" I mean both doctors and patients—are going to have to spend some time working on our partnership.

WHAT WENT WRONG?

Derailed Encounters

▼
▼

Have you ever gotten into an actual argument with your doctor? While out-and-out battles are an extreme, most of us have, at one time or another, felt dissatisfied with a visit to the doctor even though things seemed to go well on the surface. Intrinsically, the doctor–patient encounter is fraught with risks and pitfalls. All too often, both fail to realize their potential. The patient is anxious, the doctor usually isn't. The problem they are there to deal with is a personal threat to the patient and a professional challenge to the doctor. At the beginning of the visit, each has a completely different viewpoint. The perceptions and emotions they experience are very different. Their knowledge base, values, and very often their goals are different. So incongruence is inevitable.

Some problems are avoidable, others aren't. Simple things such as the physical setting, timing, and logistics of your encounter—lack of privacy, interfering noises, interruptions, schedule mix-ups—can make it impossible to succeed even when both parties are highly motivated. Perhaps a construction crew is tearing down the building next door and your few minutes with the doctor are also demolished. Or maybe the air-conditioning fails the moment you set foot in the waiting room. Most of the obstacles to success, however, have been found to lie in the actual chemistry between doctors and patients. Seventy percent, in fact.

After we leave a doctor's office, we replay the scene over and over in our heads, remembering the things we forgot to say and realizing the things we did say that might have sounded ignorant or even "stupid." It's universal. In almost every situation in life—test taking, job interviews, first dates—we become aware of everything we could have done better only after the event is over. The delayed realization that we forgot to introduce topics, make clever replies, or ask intelligent questions has been referred to by the French as the spirit of the staircase, *"esprit de l'escalier,"* which means that only as you're walking down the stairs after you've seen an important person do you remember what you had wanted to talk about.

It is because we care so much that we get nervous and insecure. We are so involved with our own anxiety, the desire to please, and the pressure of time, that we are unable to focus on the points we want to discuss. When the doctor asks what we don't know, under pressure, we come up with something. Amazingly, we even find ourselves wondering if what we told the doctor in good faith was really accurate, if we got across how bad we actually feel and why we are so worried, and if the doctor even likes us.

Do doctors like some patients more than others? Just as all of us have preferences among the people we know, so do physicians. It's not that being liked necessarily means that you're a good patient or not being liked means that you're a bad patient. One physician's favorite may be another's least liked. This may relate to the nature of the patient's complaint or the patient as a person. Sometimes it's both. In general, most doctors like to care for patients who are basically healthy and have single complaints or just one disease that the physician can treat. All doctors like to diagnose and treat illness. Some are especially gratified when they are able to diagnose complex diseases or unusual symptoms. They are programmed for success and may feel they have failed when their patients don't get well. Chronic conditions, which don't improve, frustrate them.

Doctors are less well trained to take care of patients who use sickness as a way of getting attention, as "entrance tickets" to the doctor's office. These are usually very needy people who present their doctors with numerous problems that have no medical solutions. When patients come in with constantly changing symptoms or body aches and pains for which no cause can be found, they program the doctor for failure.

It doesn't seem quite fair that when you're sick and need help that you should have to worry about how you're coming across. There are many different aspects of how we present ourselves that cause doctors to react. I remember visiting a ward at a county hospital where there were quite a few patients with cirrhosis of the liver. Most of the patients were alcoholics from disadvantaged backgrounds and were poor and uneducated. While we were on rounds one day, the supervising surgeon was taken aback by what he found on one patient's bedside table. *"How about this!"* he exclaimed, stopping in his tracks at the patient's bed. *"There aren't many patients at the county hospital who read The New Yorker!"* From that moment on, the doctors treated that patient with special consideration. For instance, when they talked to other patients, they routinely used fear tactics like,

> *"If you keep drinking like that, you'll drink yourself to death in a couple of years."*

But for the *"New Yorker"* patient, they instead stressed the positive:

> *"You still have a good portion of your liver that's well functioning, and if you stop drinking, you may do very well."*

These physicians didn't base their strategy for eliciting compliance on systematic information about the patient; instead, they were influenced by an incidental observation, a sophisticated magazine.

Within every doctor's practice, there are certain individuals who present themselves in ways that cause them to get better care. Just a moment ago, I was out in the corridor and a pediatrician was walking along, holding an exceptionally appealing baby in his arms: *"Isn't she a winner!"* he remarked, grinning ear to ear. When the next passerby offered yet another compliment, the doctor reaffirmed, *"The cutest baby in the clinic today!"* This baby aroused positive responses in everybody and that was certainly bound to influence the treatment she received. She was in a good mood and her mother presented her clean and beautifully dressed. It all helped.

All of us assess personality, attractiveness, and intelligence in the people we meet. Although going to the doctor is not a social encounter, the common rules of conduct and courtesy still apply. Dressing nicely, for instance, no matter where it is you are going, suggests that you respect the people and the occasion. This works in both directions. Have you ever felt that your doctor's attire is too casual? Does that make you wonder whether he or she is taking the encounter seriously? On the other hand, if your doctor is too proper, you may hesitate to open up on some touchy subjects. There are lots of factors—personality, setting, the situation—on both sides of the equation that may influence the medical encounter.

How to Turn Off Your Doctor in the First Five Minutes

Patients can inappropriately approach their doctors in various ways. Let's begin with thoughtless comments. Just imagine for a moment that you are on a first visit with a new doctor. You are asked why you chose this particular practice. You reply honestly with something like,

> *"The doctor I usually go to didn't have any appointments available for several weeks."*
> *"You were the closest to my job."*
> *"Because I am no longer able to see my own doctor, I lost my insurance from work."*

What this really says is, *"I didn't choose you because of your qualifications."*

If you attribute your choice simply to happenstance, it will not be the best beginning for the relationship. How would you feel, for instance, if a doctor came in to the examination room and said,

> *"I don't usually accept new patients and I'm not sure why they put you on my list, but now that you're here, we better go ahead with the examination anyway."*

It's just like going to a dinner party and saying to your hostess,

> *"I didn't have anything else to do, so I figured I might as well come."*

The cooperative effort between doctor and patient is also endangered when patients create a self-fulfilling prophesy of failure by bringing a negative attitude to the visit:

"I've already been to so many doctors with this and nobody's been able to help me. I don't suppose you will either because there probably isn't anything that will help."

Doctors, more than any other group of professionals, are success oriented. They want to win, disease is the enemy, and making people well is their goal. If you predict failure and disappointment at the start, you are putting up barriers to success.

When patients whine their way through long descriptions of symptoms, they risk losing the doctor's attention. Here, in response to the question,

"So how was your year?"

a patient told her doctor,

"I had bronchitis at the beginning of the year. It was a terrible year. God, first the bronchitis, which I had for months . . . I woke up coughing every five minutes, I didn't sleep for weeks, my throat was so dry at night and my head was exploding! Then I got the stomach flu. For a week I had nothing but diet 7-Up, and I got so weak, I couldn't get out of bed. And then someone rear-ended me on the freeway and now I have whiplash. You wouldn't believe how much it hurts. Sitting at my desk at work is pure agony."

How would you feel if you were the doctor? How would you respond? It's important for patients not to present themselves as overly helpless.

Obviously, when you go to the doctor, it's necessary to talk about what's bothering you. It's not that you shouldn't complain or say, *"I don't know what to do,"* and it's not that doctors aren't willing to listen to how much patients have suffered and need help. But when patients completely dump their problems on them, they begin to distance themselves and become less attentive. Although feelings of helplessness are not always within our control, it is important to make an effort to display as positive an attitude as possible. *"What can I do on my own to get better?"* will provide the doctor with incentive to help.

Although doctors always do have to ask a great many questions of their patients, they may react negatively when patients ask them inappropriate questions. If you pose the right questions at the right time and benefit from what the doctor says, it will, of course, further the communication. But if you ask questions or make requests that show you distrust what you're being told, you may be getting yourself into trouble. If, for example, the doctor says,

"You don't have a bacterial infection; this is a virus."

and you respond with something like,

"How do you know that, you didn't do a test."

it may not be appropriate. Your question may be intellectually justified, but if you are not in a life-and-death situation and the doctor is experienced and speaks with a certain amount of confidence, challenging him could do more harm than good. What you are really saying is,

"I don't believe you yet. Prove it to me."

to which the doctor has every right to reply:

"Okay, if it'll make you feel better, that's what we'll do. I don't think tests are necessary and they are expensive, but if that's what will do it for you, then that's what we'll do."

The doctor is now patronizing. His tone of voice and his choice of words say that he really doesn't think it's necessary.

A new patient whom I was examining recently asked,

"Are you one of the regular nurses around here?"

Barely concealing my irritation, I responded,

"I may be regular, but I'm not a nurse!"

Some patients have trouble trusting female physicians because they don't fit their image of what a doctor should look like. Sometimes, simply out of curiosity, patients ask questions that come across as challenging the physician's authenticity and credentials.

"Have you seen any cases like this before?"
"How many children have you raised?"
"Where did you go to medical school?"
"How long since you graduated?"

These challenges often come up when something unexpected happens, or the doctor makes a comment such as,

"Oh, I've never seen that before."

You might think it's unrealistic for a patient to trust a doctor up front without doing some double-checking, but once you have chosen someone and are there for a consultation, it's not the time to open a negotiation about credentials.

What does it do to the therapeutic alliance if you bring a relative or friend with you to the appointment or you are accompanied by someone? Teenage girls often bring girlfriends in to the office with them to serve as protection, which makes it very hard for the doctor to establish a relationship. Older patients may be driven to the doctor by a concerned relative who, with the best of intentions, may accompany the patient throughout the visit. This carries the risk of transforming the patient into the object of the discussion rather than an active participant. When couples come in together and the doctor begins trying to negotiate health care with the one who is his patient, it can prove difficult when the other person starts giving opinions and making suggestions.

The doctor–patient encounter, by definition, should be confidential and that's not easy when other participants are present. When members of a family go to the same doctor, complicated situations can arise. Suppose one person becomes concerned about another and wants to talk to the doctor privately. It may be difficult to do so without the other person finding out. A teenager, for instance, wishes to discuss family planning with her doctor but has not yet confessed to her parents that she is sexually active. She finds it impossible to talk to her doctor because her mother always accompanies her into the examination room.

Patients bring people along for a number of reasons—for support, for protection, and sometimes simply because they like to have company. But for the doctor who is trying to create a relationship, the extra person can become an unwelcome intrusion, a "bodyguard" who comes between him and the patient. How would you feel if the doctor asked the nurse to be present during the entire visit when you were expecting to have a private conversation? It's always hard to talk to more than one person at a time. Think about the last instance you had a telephone conversation and someone in the room began talking while you were trying to listen to another person through the receiver. Not only is it difficult to hear, but it becomes nearly impossible to establish a relationship with either participant. It's up to the physician and the patient to choose when it's necessary to involve other people and when they need to be alone. Although at times you may wish to invite others to accompany you, be careful not to establish a routine that precludes adequate private time.

Another frequent error is for patients to think they can ingratiate themselves with the doctors they are currently consulting by criticizing other doctors or medical personnel:

"This is the best exam I've ever had; my other doctor never had me undress . . . ."

A patient I saw the other day became effusive in telling me how wonderful I was only after stating,

"I'm glad they didn't assign me to that young Dr. Jones today. He really doesn't have the necessary experience. I like someone who has a few gray hairs like you and I know you're the only one who can give me any answers."

My heart sank. Physicians do not welcome this approach. They tend to see it as a ploy and it arouses their suspicions—*How long will it be before she says the same things about me?*

Just think about other life situations. If, for example, you are at a social gathering and someone makes a negative statement about all women—

"You know how women are, they never can get ready on time"—

every woman in that room will bristle. Or imagine yourself dining in a restaurant with someone who says,

"Someone else I recently dined with was really hard to talk to."

You might begin to worry that your dinner partner might soon become critical of you as a conversationalist. Similarly, when most experienced doctors hear patients blame others, they realize that it won't be long before they themselves come under fire.

Other idle comments about doctors will also cause trouble:

"Doctors never listen."
"Doctors are always in a hurry."
"When you go to the doctor, you always have to wait."

Any one of those statements is likely to erect a barrier, especially in a new relationship. Every physician functions not only as an individual but also as a conscientious representative of the medical profession. Yet each of us wants a chance to present ourselves as we are and not be categorized on the basis of what others have done. This is true in almost any human context. If you go out on a date and say, *"I distrust good looking men because the ones I've seen always turn out to be vain,"* you are making a negative generalization about a group of people that may not apply to your escort, even if he is devastatingly handsome.

Another inappropriate strategy is for patients to try to influence their doctor's treatment or diagnosis by giving anecdotal experiences from other people and other doctors:

"I know someone who had the same exact thing and what they did was . . . ."

The big problem is that by relating the anecdotes of neighbors, friends, or relatives, patients are making loose generalizations. For instance, suppose that your child is having trouble sleeping and you consult a doctor. If the doctor responds with, *"Whenever my child had trouble going to sleep, all I did was let him cry it out for three nights and we had no further problems,"* you may find yourself without a satisfactory solution. The two situations involve completely different people and circumstances. So if you begin talking about cousin Joe's similar problems and how he solved them, don't expect a warm reaction. Whenever you get sick, suddenly everyone you know has had "the same thing":

"I had back pain just like that last year and what I did was . . . ."
"I had the same flu symptoms and what I did was . . . ."
"You know what I've found helps my migraines is . . . ."

Just as we become exasperated by the stories and opinions around us, doctors also get sick of hearing about Aunt Tilly or Uncle Roger who had *exactly* the same thing. What our doctors want is information about our own health.

If you, as a patient, have experienced a similar situation before, it might be appropriate to say something to the effect,

"The last time I coughed like this, it turned out that I had a secondary infection in my sinuses—do you think that might be what's going on with me now?"

Or, if you are coming down with the flu and are aware that other people at work have had similar symptoms, then that's information that may help your doctor. Talk about yourself and your symptoms. Ask general questions for information, but don't insist that because you know that penicillin helped somebody else that it is the right treatment for you.

What about patients who are well read? Physicians do advocate patient education by means of reading, listening to the media, and taking advantage of materials available in the office. Yet patients sometimes get into trouble when they misinterpret acquired information or introduce it at an inappropriate time. If you find something while reading that seems contrary to what the doctor said and you challenge:

> *"You told me that I should put cold packs on when I tore my ligaments, but this booklet says that warm is much better, it improves the circulation!"*

that's picking a fight. Try saying instead,

> *"I hope you'll understand. I found a book on this which says that after I use cold packs for the first twenty-four hours to reduce the swelling, it's a good idea to put on warm compresses. Do you think that would work for me?"*

If you introduce new information in an open-minded way, most doctors should be willing to discuss it. But if you spend too much time talking about what you've learned through other sources instead of benefiting from what your doctor can tell you, you're making poor use of the time.

A friend of mine who has chronic fatigue syndrome, a rare disease that some doctors don't even consider a "real" physical disease, was consistently put off by her doctors when she asked for further reading. In desperation, she went on the Internet and sent out a request for information. She received an extraordinary number of responses from people with the same symptoms—some with useful advice, some not. She then began to worry about how to approach her doctors, and because she had already implemented some of the advice, she ended up too afraid and embarrassed to mention it at all.

As you might imagine, taking a stack of information into a doctor's office may not be very welcome. Whether you obtain your information from the library, television, or the Internet, keep in mind that no two cases are alike, it's probably not a simple subject, and you may end up more confused than educated. Think about what you want from your doctor in relation to the information. Avoid a *Look what I know and you don't* attitude. Ideally, your doctor will be able to clarify the information for you. Prioritize. Don't try to cover too much, and concentrate on the most important issues you'd like to know more about.

What do doctors think about alternative treatments? Especially in the cases of patients who have severe or even life-threatening diseases, doctors need to be open-minded and sensitive enough to realize that those people are desperate and will try anything. But it's also important for patients to realize that doctors become frustrated when they have no effective treatments to offer, and so when patients then propose treatments that make no medical sense, doctors tend to get angry:

> *"A friend brought me an herb tea from China that's been shown to cure many cases of cancer."*

Misguided hopes for cures and treatment hoaxes spring up for almost every disease. The more desperate patients are, the more prone they are to want to try things. Sadly, it is often the patients with severe diseases such as cancer who become the victims of irresponsible entrepreneurs who offer alternate treatments.

In pediatric practice, we see a great many parents put effort and hope into useless treatment interventions for their developmentally disabled children. Some years ago the physicians at a well-known clinic in Philadelphia developed a treatment plan that they believed would accelerate the development of retarded children. The treatment itself was harmless and consisted of a series of exercises that recapitulated developmental phases. Children were taught how to crawl and were put through other bodily motions that simulated what would happen in normal development. On careful follow-up, however, it became apparent that the treatments produced no significant progress.[1] Although the experience did no harm to any of the children, the fact that the parents were given false hope led many to spend their life savings, and disrupt their daily family life to make the trip to Philadelphia, all in the vain hope that it might help their children.

Whenever the families of retarded patients I was taking care of got discouraged and said, *"We're going to Philadelphia for those special treatments,"* I became truly exasperated. It was upsetting to see them succumb to these misleading claims. Although I tried to explain that it would be a waste of their time and effort, they dismissed me as defensive about my own performance.

Physicians may not react positively when patients consult alternative healers, practitioners, or even physicians abroad. In certain areas, pharmaceutical substances are less carefully controlled than they are in the United States. For instance, cortisone and some antibiotics are given out much more freely than they are in our own communities. Suppose you are the doctor. Would you want a patient who is taking something that you feel may be putting him at risk? After all, you are now responsible. You might not know exactly what the medication is or whether it could be harmful.

We videotaped a doctor in the cardiology clinic who asked his patient if she had been taking "her medicine." There were two or three medications she was supposed to be taking, and when she began digging in her purse to find them, she brought out about six or seven additional bottles she had gotten in another country. A typical response would have been for the doctor to make disparaging remarks:

> *"I don't care what that doctor prescribed for you, what you need are the medications I prescribed the last time and I don't want you to take anything else!"*

Luckily for this patient, her doctor was open-minded and commented:

> *"You seem to have a few more medications there than we prescribed for you."*

She explained that she got them in Mexico and that her relatives had told her to go there to consult a doctor.

"Well, let's look and see what these are," he said, and then began looking at each one, explaining what they might or might not do. At the end of the visit, even though he found that she did not require any of these additional medications, his attitude was so accepting and nonjudgmental that it was possible for them to continue working together.

If you are interested in pursuing an alternate course of treatment, it would be wise to discuss it with your primary doctor. You need to find out whether there's anything about that treatment that he thinks might be harmful. Remember, the treatment may have worked for someone else, but you are a completely different patient. The physician's reaction will depend on the severity of the disease, the nature of the treatment, and the likelihood that it could do harm.

When Patient's Concerns Aren't Heard

One of the most common problems is that patients feel their doctors never understood their main concerns. In my initial studies, about three-quarters of patients felt that their main concerns had never been heard and responded to.[2] This predictably derails the patient in his or her efforts to communicate with the doctor.

The mother in the following excerpt is completely at odds with her doctor. They spent over forty minutes together, and both ended up completely frustrated. She had taken her daughter to an emergency facility the night before with a high temperature and what she believed was a rapid heartbeat.

> DOCTOR: *Did they take her temperature at the Emergency Hospital last night?*
>
> MOTHER: *Yeah.*
>
> DOCTOR: *Now, what symptoms has she been having besides this feeling warm at night?*
>
> MOTHER: *Well, that's it! That's why . . . .*
>
> DOCTOR: (Interrupts) *She feels fine.*
>
> MOTHER: *In the daytime!*

The mother's frustration begins when the doctor does not seem to acknowledge her daughter's symptoms and also constantly interrupts her.

> DOCTOR: *Hmmm . . . . How does she feel at night?*
>
> MOTHER: *You ask her how she feels right now and Maria will tell you she feels fine but later . . . .*

DOCTOR: (Interrupts) *What about at night?*

MOTHER: *She'll tell you fine but she can't be—*

DOCTOR: (Interrupts) *Hmm . . . now . . . does she complain of anything?*

MOTHER: *No, that's what—uh fooled me, you know what I mean because . . . I ask, "Maria does your throat hurt?" "No." "Does your stomach hurt?" "No." You know, so I don't know what it is, doctor, but I know her heart, maybe if you listen . . . . It doesn't sound normal. It is just beating too fast. And one night when Maria says, "Mother, hold my hand, I'm lonely" you know right there something's wrong. She's never done that before. I hope it's nothing serious. I'll make myself sick. All I need is a kid with a heart condition. I'm a nervous mother, if you know what that is. No good, huh? I'm 46 and she's 6. Now doctor, don't say she hasn't got a heart murmur. I can hear it myself . . . .*

DOCTOR: *There is nothing wrong with this child's heart. You have a very healthy girl here.*

MOTHER: *She doesn't look right . . . .*

CHILD: *You got fooled, Mama!*

MOTHER: *Well . . . Maria has a more vivacious look, you know.*

The doctor says the child is fine. The mother says she isn't, but can't come up with any specifics. In the meantime, the child, who perceives the doctor's attitude, also turns against her mother. The mother is doubly invalidated.

DOCTOR: *Yeah. I would suggest that you either buy a thermometer and learn how to read it . . . .*

MOTHER: *I . . . .*

DOCTOR: *. . . or else stop feeling her forehead at night, unless she complains of feeling sick, because you cannot tell what a child's temperature is just by feeling.*

MOTHER: (Interrupts) *No, I can't tell what it is, but I can tell if she is running a fever.*

In a patronizing and condescending tone, the doctor debunks this mother's observations and deprecates her skills in caring for her child. Without exploring any further, he assumes that she does not have a thermometer when, in fact, it was found later that she did have one but felt, as many mothers do, that she could tell whether her child had a fever.

DOCTOR: *Well, if you think she's running a fever, you should take her temperature then. Buy yourself a thermometer and learn how to read it. Then, if she is running a high temperature, have her checked at that time. She has absolutely no temperature at this time.*

MOTHER: *No! She don't have it except at night!*

The mother still believes that the doctor is unaware of the seriousness of her child's condition and is unable to accept his reassurance.

DOCTOR: *Well, I don't hear anything wrong with her heart at all and I would let her go to school and she's a perfectly normal child and you can't tell anything by listening like that.*

MOTHER: *No, but I just wondered, that's all. I don't know . . . doctor, you think I'm gonna come over here this morning. It scared me half to death when I got a report like this!*

DOCTOR: *Well, I think she's a normal child and I would let her go to school and I wouldn't worry about her.*

MOTHER: *Forget it, huh? Okay, Maria.*

When she left, the mother had given up any hope of engaging the doctor. After a lengthy visit, nothing had been accomplished. The mother did not believe that the doctor understood, and she ended up seeking out another doctor. The physician, meanwhile, writes off his patient as uncooperative.

In this next excerpt, another mother is so insistent about not keeping her child at home that she quickly turns her doctor against the idea that her son should be hospitalized. She feels as if she has failed to get her message across and, in turn, that the doctor has let her down.

DOCTOR: *OK . . . well, he still has pneumonia clinically . . . . I hear a pneumonia. Sometimes you can hear it, but it doesn't show up on the X ray for twenty-four hours. So I'll go ahead and give him penicillin.*

MOTHER: *So, he must be starting to get it. M-hm.* (Anxiously) *Aren't you going to hospitalize him?*

DOCTOR: (Matter-of-fact) *He doesn't need to be hospitalized.*

MOTHER: *Ooooh, Doctor! I'm going to have a hard time keeping him down in our house . . . it's so old and drafty.*

DOCTOR: *M-hm. Well, he can walk around. He doesn't have to go to bed.*

MOTHER: *Can he?*

DOCTOR: *Sure.*

MOTHER: *But . . . last night, when he got so awfully hot . . . what do you do when he gets the tremor . . . you know . . . he had 104 yesterday. I thought that was pretty high.*

DOCTOR: *Yeah, well, we'll see him back in one week and get another chest X ray to be sure nothing's there.*

MOTHER: *M-hm.*

DOCTOR: *Okay?*

MOTHER: *You think he's nothing to worry about?*

DOCTOR: *It's nothing serious.*

MOTHER: *Nothing serious.*

DOCTOR: *But don't let him go outside. Keep him in the house. He can run around. He doesn't have to stay in bed. M-hm. Okay?*

MOTHER: (Interrupts) *And he really runs . . . he just tears through the house.*

DOCTOR: *That's okay. So come up to the front desk and they'll give you . . . .*

MOTHER: *Nothing special to eat?*

DOCTOR: *No.*

MOTHER: *Juices?*

DOCTOR: *Anything he wants . . . lots of juices.*

FATHER: *I mean, let him play around?*

DOCTOR: *He can play around. It would be easier to let him play than keep him in bed.*

MOTHER: *M-hm. It's awfully hard to keep him down. If he's upstairs, he's got to stay in bed or else go in the hospital.*

DOCTOR: *No, he doesn't have to be in the hospital.*

MOTHER: *Uh . . . it is because they are short of beds upstairs, may I ask . . . or what?*

DOCTOR: *No. We don't usually hospitalize pneumonia.*

MOTHER: *Don't you anymore?*

DOCTOR: *No.*

MOTHER: *Uh . . . what kind of pneumonia is that, would you say? What was it he had before this?*

FATHER: *Bronchial.*

MOTHER: *Bronchial?*

FATHER: *Bronchial.*

MOTHER: *Lobar?*

DOCTOR: *Bronchial . . . it's the same thing.*

MOTHER: *Is that what it is, bronchial now?*

DOCTOR: *M-hm.*

MOTHER: *Okey-doke. No more X rays, did you say . . . today?*

DOCTOR: *Not today.*

MOTHER: *I see. Well, thank you.*

The doctor leaves the room. Even though these parents did not hesitate to ask questions, the mother is furious and completely unsatisfied with the doctor:

MOTHER: (Talking to father) *I think he should be hospitalized! And
     I'm his mother! And I've been around him more than five minutes!
     I'm his mother! I'm the one who has to treat him!*

Although she stressed that her son's fever was so high that he got "tremors," this mother's concerns were dismissed. She is frightened because she sees pneumonia as a very serious disease that requires hospitalization. Having to wait one week to be seen again gives her little comfort. The physician, as so often is the case, speaks strictly from a medical point of view. Saying that he "hears a pneumonia" and that sometimes it "doesn't show up on the X ray for twenty-four hours" are technical details that mean little to the mother. When the doctor states that he is not going to put the child in the hospital, she thinks that he doesn't recognize how serious her son's condition is and begins to insist again how sick her son really is. The parents make repeated attempts to learn what kind of pneumonia their child has,

*"What kind of pneumonia is that, would you say? What was it he
had before this? . . . Bronchial ? . . . Lobar?"*
but they are told vaguely,
" . . . it's the same thing."

For all of us, just having a name for what's wrong gives us a sense of mastery. The parents would have felt better if they at least had a name to attach to the illness.

Neither partner helped the cooperative venture along. The mother made a strategic error by suggesting hospitalization before the child's illness had been fully explained. Telling a doctor what to do is always risky and, in this case, it certainly proved to be a turnoff. In return, the doctor failed to enlist the mother's cooperation, never making sure that she knew that he understood her concerns. He gave no advice as to how to care for the child and simply told her to go home. The doctor's entire demeanor suggests that he might have been thinking that the mother was unwilling to take the responsibility of caring for her child at home. What didn't get enough emphasis and should have is that penicillin can cure pneumonia. Had he been sensitive to the situation, he might have told her that, in former years, pneumonia meant hospitalization, but reassured her that today there is a very effective treatment.

When Patients Expect the Impossible

When patients come in with unrealistic expectations, the doctor is frustrated right from the start and satisfying the patient becomes difficult, if not impossible. Many patients think that when they go to specialists—whether dermatologists, gynecologists, or orthopedists—that they should be able to help with unrelated problems as well. Will your internist be upset if you ask for a Pap smear when you have your annual checkup? Can you ask your gynecologist about your headaches or will he suggest that you discuss this with your family doctor? What if you think you are coming down with the flu when you see your dermatologist? Can you ask for treatment? Generally, it's better not to burden doctors with complaints that are not in their area of expertise or ask them for prescriptions for conditions they did not diagnose. A patient who goes to her annual gynecological appointment and asks for antibiotics because she has a terribly sore throat will actually be imposing because her request is not within her doctor's delineated area of responsibility. If he does not look at her throat and suggests she go to her primary physician, he may begin to worry later:

> *"Maybe I should have done a throat culture right then and there. What if she really gets sick?"*

Worse yet, the patient may later hold him responsible.

Another patient is seeing her orthopedist on a follow-up visit for a sports injury and, as he is finishing the exam, she says,

> *"Oh, I almost forgot, my primary care doctor always gives me a prescription for Valium but I'm not due to see her for another two months. Could you do it for me?"*

This really puts him on the spot.

Sometimes patients ask for help with family conflicts without realizing that they are requesting the impossible:

> *"Please talk to my son and make him stop talking back to his father."*
> *"I want you to talk to my husband about his drinking."*

These are things for which your doctor cannot take responsibility. Of course, there are times when another family member's behavior directly affects your health and, in those cases, you are justified in asking your doctor to become involved. If you have an ulcer, for instance, and your husband continues to insist on meals that are bad for your stomach, then it wouldn't be out-of-line to request,

> *"My husband always wants me to cook rich dinners and I remember that you told me it's not good for my condition. Would it be possible for the three of us to have a conference?"*

Doctors get frustrated when you ask for things they can't deliver. Amazingly, patients sometimes expect their doctors to know what's wrong without even telling them. In this next excerpt from a videotaped encounter, a mother who has brought her child in for an examination literally tests the physician by refusing to give him the information he asks for.

DOCTOR: *What's wrong with his gait?*

MOTHER: *Huh?*

DOCTOR: *What . . . what don't you like about the way he walks?*

MOTHER: *Well he falls all the time. His leg is just . . . it's constantly giving out on him.*

DOCTOR: *Which leg?*

MOTHER: *I want _you_ to find out which leg.*

DOCTOR: *No, you tell _me_. I want to know what the story is.*

MOTHER: *I'm supposed to tell _you_? You're not supposed to find out any-thing?*

DOCTOR: *Well, I mean . . . .*

MOTHER: *Well.*

DOCTOR: *I mean that's like looking for something in a haystack. If you won't tell me what the problem is.*

MOTHER: *I don't know the problem. That's what I came here for!*

The mother stubbornly refused to give the information, feeling that it was the doctor's job to make the diagnosis. She wanted the doctor to prove his competence and therefore he should have been able to find out on his own. This made the doctor angry because he felt it was her job to supply a certain amount of the information. The visit continued to slide downhill from there.

Sometimes patients do not deliberately withhold information, but are unable to remember everything the doctor is asking for. An acquaintance, Julie, told me about what had happened when her husband Ted went to see the doctor. They made the appointment because Ted was having breathing difficulties at night. Julie had accompanied her husband to the doctor's office and had naturally expected that she would remain in the waiting area. But when the doctor asked Ted at what time in the night he was troubled by wheezing and he couldn't remember exactly, the doctor then called Julie into the examination room. She was able to supply all the necessary infor-mation. While it was a prudent move on the doctor's part, Julie thought it was unusual that it was she who was giving the history on Ted's behalf. And Ted felt embarrassed that he hadn't been able to remember and was uncom-fortable with the fact that his wife had to provide the information. The cou-ple left the office feeling somewhat inadequate and that they hadn't come across very well.

There are many reasons why you may not be able to come up with the information the doctor requests. If you are in a social situation and some-one asks you something trivial that you can't remember,

"When did you have dinner with the Joneses?"

and you have to turn to your spouse to inquire,

"Dear, was it last Wednesday or Thursday?"

that doesn't make you feel bad. But if your doctor requests information:

> *"Exactly when did you first notice that your headaches were getting more severe?"*
> *"Can you remember the first time you noticed blurred vision?"*
> *"In the past couple of months, how often have you noticed the numbness and tingling in your hand?"*

and you're not able to come up with it, you feel inadequate.

Actually, the doctor might think you were overanxious, too compulsive, and perhaps even suspect you of being a hypochondriac if you rushed in with a list of days and times when you did have blurred vision. It's human to be bothered by symptoms, but not to count and date them. Of course, if the doctor asks you to keep a detailed record for the next time, that's another story. When you have not been able to come up with information quickly and completely enough, it may cause you to feel that the doctor didn't really understand your concerns. At that point it's up to you to speak up and let the doctor know. If you remember something after the visit, you should call your doctor's office and tell the receptionist or assistant that you have remembered something that the doctor had asked for.

You may also be expecting the impossible if you ask doctors to do things that they cannot do in good conscience. In my own experience, social acquaintances and friends often ask me to sign prescriptions for sedatives or other medicines. When I decline, they let me know how annoyed they are.

> *"Why are you doctors so fussy about signing prescriptions? All you have to do is sign your name! I'm only going to get a few pills—they are not going to do me any harm. My other doctor never had a problem with giving them to me."*

It's hard for a patient to understand why this is an unrealistic expectation; doctors should not sign prescriptions unless they have examined the patient themselves. Sometimes patients call on the phone and want refills for medication when the doctor hasn't seen them for a long time and does not know whether it is still necessary. They may think that they are saving the doctor some time, but they are actually putting the doctor on the spot. In this next excerpt, a patient pleads with her doctor for a higher dosage of medication than he originally prescribed.

"I just can't function without my Darvocet . . . at home it's like a circus, it's always noisy and nobody ever listens to me . . . and Sally, well, you know what teenagers are like. Her high school is in a bad neighborhood where there's a lot of gang activity. I try to sleep but I can't. Those sick headaches of mine are so terrible that I can hardly get up in the morning. I really need some relief. I have too much pain . . . .

You've given me my prescription before. I don't know why you won't do it now. And the last one wasn't even enough to help. Maybe you could give me something stronger."

People frequently ask their doctors to do things that are unethical, sometimes even illegal. Doctors are commonly asked to give false information on insurance forms, get unjustified handicapped parking permits, fabricate excuses for not going to work. Years ago, the only way a pregnant woman could have a legal abortion was to obtain reports from two physicians who had examined her and made a diagnosis of German measles. The reason for this was that German measles in the first trimester of pregnancy can cause severe abnormalities in the fetus. So, not infrequently, women who were distressed about being pregnant would request physicians to sign certificates saying that they had German measles. These patients actually counted on their doctors to lie for them. They would complain,

"All you have to do is sign it! I don't understand why you won't do that for me. If you don't, I don't know what I'm going to do."

Even though a doctor might have been deeply moved by a young woman's plight, as an honest doctor he could not sign such a statement.

Another issue that puts doctors on the spot is when patients make misleading promises on their behalf. In pediatrics, it infuriates us when we hear a mother tell a crying child,

"If you stop crying, the doctor won't give you any shots today."

Or, worse yet,

"If you don't behave, I'm going to tell the doctor to keep you here!"

On the one hand, we don't want the child to feel that we are breaking a promise if we do have to give an injection, and, on the other, we don't want to make the mother look bad in front of the child. Similarly, if a patient goes to a doctor and says, *"I recommended you to my sister. I told her that you were the only one who cured my migraines and that you'd be the one who would do it for her too,"* even though the patient thinks the doctor will be pleased by the confidence she has shown him, he finds himself uneasy. He has no idea why his new patient is getting headaches and is unsure whether he will actually be able to help her.

Don't waste time and effort trying to get the doctor to fix things that are out of his control. Every day, for example, patients complain about how long it takes to get through on the switchboard,

"I've tried for a week to get through."
"The lines are always busy."
"I was so sick! I couldn't stay on hold forever!"
"That operator of yours was so rude to me!"
"How can I make an appointment if I can't get through?"

Believe it or not, your doctor is probably just as exasperated, if not more so, than you are. You're spending time that might be used to better advantage; the doctor probably can't change the switchboard operator and has a limited amount of time to spend with you. A few years ago, I learned this lesson firsthand when I landed in the hospital for surgery. The housekeeping services were grossly inadequate—in fact my room had not been thoroughly cleaned for several days. When my doctor came by on rounds, I immediately confronted him with,

"Look, something should be done about this. The place is filthy!"

Controlling his irritation, he replied,

"Everybody's annoyed with the fact that it isn't very clean here, but it isn't something I have any control over. I have to see all my patients in the morning before I go to surgery and the time I spend discussing cleaning takes away from the time I have to care for patients."

So it doesn't make much sense to spend both our energy and the doctor's time on things they cannot change. If you walked into an examination room and the doctor complained to you, *"Too many patients come in here who haven't got their insurance cards and don't have the necessary forms. It sure makes it so difficult for us,"* you would probably get impatient. Those are things you cannot help. You would probably prefer to spend the time concentrating on your own problems.

If you make your doctor responsible for everything that's wrong with the system—billing practices, housecleaning, the switchboard, long waits, and so on—you are misusing your own time and power. If you can avoid complaining to the doctor about irrelevant matters, do so. The best thing to do is to find out on your own who is accountable. Ask the receptionist:

"Who around here is in charge of the telephone operation? Someone was really rude to me."

Nowadays, we are all living under such a bureaucracy that, even though doctors used to be the top of the hierarchy, you can no longer assume that they have control.

It is not realistic to expect your doctor to deal with all your medical problems as well as those afflicting other members of your family. Predictably, if you start mentioning one problem after another, the doctor will begin to worry. One of our interns presented the case of a little girl, age five, who had a complicated history of earaches. She'd had an earache in one ear, then the other, then both, and then they went away. Sometimes there was a fever with it, sometimes there wasn't. The intern had examined her ears and found nothing wrong, but her parents were certain there was. They had consulted several specialists without results. After listening to this complex and sometimes inconsistent set of complaints, I began to question whether we could possibly be of any help. When I went into the examination room with the intern, I noticed the mother herself had a little bit of cotton in her ear.

> *"Well, I've been having trouble with my ear," she began. "And I have a relative who has deafness in one ear and . . . ."*

At that point, we became discouraged because we had been presented with too many problems. It was a setup for disappointment because we failed to find anything wrong with the child's ear and on top of that were confronted with the mother's own ear problem.

What, then, do you do if you have more than one problem you'd like to talk about? Most patients do. First, remember that there are limitations to what can be accomplished. Try to establish some priorities. For which of your problems do you need the most help? What do you find the most disturbing? Be ready to have your priorities dictate what you will emphasize without omitting to mention the others. The doctor might not be able to respond to all of them. It's a good idea to let your doctor know that you understand this:

> *"I know this isn't what I came in for but I wanted to let you know about it. If there's not enough time today, perhaps I could schedule another appointment to talk about it?"*

While you should make sure the doctor has heard about the things that are bothering you because they may add up to something, don't expect to walk in with three problems and walk out with solutions to them all:

> *"For your fast heartbeat, I'm going to give you this medicine; for your constipation, I'm going to give you that; and for the headaches that keep coming up, this is the medicine that will fix it."*

You can help your doctor develop priorities that match your own by explaining what bothers you most and letting him know that you understand that not everything can be handled all in one visit.

Boundaries

Your doctor probably calls you by your first name. Have you ever called your doctor by his or her first name? Even in social situations, doctors often bristle when they are introduced as Mr. or Ms. Rightly or wrongly, they feel that it's up to them to establish the ground rules for the relationship and keep it from getting too informal. At almost every seminar on the doctor–patient relationship, physicians ask what they should do when patients unexpectedly address them by their first names. My advice has always been to take the first opportunity to say,

"Please call me Dr. . . ."

Is this a power play? Not necessarily. Physicians do have to ask very personal questions and patients need to be able to discuss intimate details without being embarrassed. In a professional relationship in which there is social distance, this is easier, but if the relationship changes into a personal one, it becomes difficult. There are some physicians who are perfectly happy and even prefer to be on a first-name basis with their patients. It may be prudent to wait until the doctor suggests such a basis:

"Please call me Jane."

While patients sometimes initiate the uninvited use of first names to the doctor's dismay, they are not the only offenders. Gynecologists, for instance, are notorious for greeting patients who are already undressed and in the embarrassing examination position,

"Hi there, Sue! How's it going?"

Or, worse yet, they give a playful slap on the patient's behind. Physicians who take care of older patients are also at risk. A heartfelt complaint on the part of many geriatric patients is that their doctors automatically talk down to them and, in fact, may use the equivalent of baby talk, often using their first names without even asking. Imagine the dignified, seventy-five-year-old grandmother whose thirty-five-year-old-yuppie doctor strolls in with a casual,

"Hello there, Mary, you're looking prettier and younger every day. What can we do for you today?"

Nursing staff frequently believe they can improve relationships with their patients by using first names. During a support group meeting for an intensive-care-unit staff, a team of concerned nurses discussed the relationships they were having with their desperately ill patients. They mentioned proudly that they had maintained a friendly atmosphere in the unit and called all their patients by their first names. When asked if there had ever been a patient who didn't like it, one nurse mentioned a judge who had been uncomfortable and had requested that he be addressed as "Your Honor." We challenged the group with a question:

"If the patient had been a garbage collector, would he have had the nerve to request that they call him by his last name?"

Although they couldn't answer, it did make them think.

A black nurse with whom I worked for a long time later told me a poignant story about her father, who had been admitted to a prominent southern medical center some years ago. This was when black patients were carefully segregated from whites, had separate wards and bathrooms, and staff were encouraged to call them by their first names. As an elderly man who wanted respect, her father had been deeply offended when he was addressed simply as "Bill." He well remembered the bad old days in the South when no black man was addressed as "Mr." and he had reached a point in his life when that was no longer acceptable. He corrected the nurse with, *"Don't call me Bill,"* and his daughter followed suit by insisting, *"His name is Mr. Washington."*

Gift-giving is another controversial ploy in the patient's approach to the doctor. Have you ever given your doctor a gift or offered a favor?

"I can arrange to get you front-row tickets for opening night."
"How about some 50-yard-line tickets?"

Such overtures come off as psychological bribes and rarely go over well. Executives and other professionals who are used to being in charge sometimes do this because they become uncomfortable when they realize that the doctor is really the one holding the reins, making the rules.

Gifts can be interpreted in many different ways. Think about the way you feel when someone you don't really know, perhaps someone you are only slightly acquainted with through work, unexpectedly gives you something. You end up feeling that you now owe them something special in return. That's how gifts from patients have always made me feel, except when it was an appropriate thoughtful gesture such as a tin of homemade cookies during the holidays or a seasonal card. But if it's something inappropriately generous, I feel uncomfortable. After all, I am doing my job. I have also found generous gifts make me feel excessively guilty when things don't go well for the patient, or if I have to give bad news. And if they ask a favor, I feel almost obligated. Although many doctors feel that way, it varies with the physician's personality and the circumstances.

One very busy, active New York physician practiced like an old country doctor. Lots of barter trade. He did things for patients and patients did things for him. During Christmas, his house was full of lavish gifts of all kinds. And then when patients needed him to tell a white lie on an insurance form or wanted a house call at an impossible hour, they felt free to ask for it and he complied. In his particular case, the gift-giving fulfilled a mutual need, but he also ended up feeling obliged to perform inappropriate services for patients.

Don't let yourself get into a power play with your doctor. A physician peremptorily instructed his patient, a busy attorney, *"On this new medication, you will have to come in every week so we can monitor your blood pressure,"* without exploring his schedule or other obligations. Insulted that the physician had not respected his work schedule, the patient responded resentfully, *"Well, you know, I'm busy too. I'm a $400-per-hour attorney and I can't really afford to spend this kind of time unless it's absolutely necessary."* This was his attempt to let it be known that his time was more valuable than that of the physician. Instead of exchanging useful information, the conversation became a competition for who was more important. If the doctor tells you to do something that you feel is unreasonable, don't get into an argument. Try to reach a negotiating position so that your ideas can move toward a solution, not an impasse. The doctor, of course, did need to hear that the proposed schedule was going to be hard for his patient. And they needed to work out a feasible plan together, without having the patient push the prestige of his position and high income. The attorney could have gotten the same point across without causing friction:

> *"I know you need to check my blood pressure regularly, but I'm not sure how I'm going to be able to rearrange my schedule. Is there any other way we could work it out?"*

In the midst of a busy office visit, some patients try to involve the doctor in irrelevant conversation:

> *"Do you think SoAndSo is guilty or innocent?"*

Or about their private lives. A patient was late for her appointment and tried to explain by saying,

> *"I'm sorry I'm late. I have a little old car that keeps breaking down."*

The doctor's terse response:

> *"I manage to keep on schedule and I expect my patients to do the same. Otherwise my office routine really suffers."*

The patient, now a little annoyed, replied,

> *"But then you probably drive a better car that doesn't break down. What kind is it?"*

She was defending herself but it got her into more trouble. His response:

> *"I presume you're not here to discuss what kind of a car I drive. What can I help you with today?"*

This doctor later told me,

> *"Her comment about the kind of car I drive made me feel as if I earn my money by taking it from poor sick people."*

For doctors on tight time schedules, unnecessary questions take up precious time that could be better spent—on you.

Asking the appropriate questions, however, is essential. Don't be afraid! A group of trainee physicians was recently in my office viewing a videotape we had made of their visits. One of their patients, a pony-tailed Hollywood musician, was extraordinarily well informed and asked a lot of questions. He told the doctor that he had been using a number of herbs and even brought along two samples of what he was currently taking. He had strong ideas about medicines and challenged the doctor on several points. One of the doctors in our group asked the physician in the video about whether he was put off by such an "opinionated" patient. The doctor responded,

> *"No, I like that kind of patient. I like someone who asks those kinds of questions because then I can tell where I am and when I'm getting across. I don't like it when a patient is too quiet or subdued."*

So typically there were doctors in our group who felt both ways: some admitted they thought he asked too many questions, others liked his openness.

Unfortunately, patients are often afraid to ask questions for fear physicians will feel challenged. Or that the doctor will think they are ignorant. For heaven's sakes, don't let the fact that some of your questions are indeed challenging scare you away from asking them. The message is to think about the intent of your questions before you ask them. Are you asking because you don't believe what the doctor is saying or doing? Or is it because you really need more information? If so, don't hesitate to make it clear that that is why you are asking. If the doctor is not able to answer all your questions or is pressed for time, which is what so many patients complain about, ask where you can get the information.

> *"Is there something I can read? Could you recommend a brochure that would be helpful?"*

In all human relationships, expressions of confidence and trust are essential. Yet patients sometimes fail to recognize the doctor as a human being who also profits from the positive aspects of the relationship. While you shouldn't flatter or make empty compliments, making positive state-ments may be helpful. Expressing your appreciation without being unduly effusive can provide a boost. If the doctor can't come up with a diagnosis and has expressed frustration by saying,

> *"I really wish I knew more about what we're dealing with but I can't tell you at this moment,"*

there is no harm in responding with,

> *"Well, I don't expect you to always know everything; nobody does. But it is good to know you're there for me and just talking to you has made me feel better."*

If you express the positive, you have also set the stage to negotiate other things more effectively. It may make you more comfortable and allow you to express criticisms and ask questions that are important to you:

> *"I know you can't possibly give me the answer today, but there are a couple of things you might be able to explain if you have another minute . . . ."*

This would then enable you to ask another question:

> *"For the next couple of weeks, what do you think I have to look forward to?"*

What About Second Opinions?

Patients hesitate to ask for second opinions because they feel uncomfortable and don't want to hurt doctors' feelings. One sure way to annoy a doctor is to get another opinion without telling him or her. Eventually, you end up back in the doctor's office saying,

> *"Well, I consulted Dr. SoAndSo and she said . . . ."*

While you may be trying to maintain a good relationship, you may actually be threatening it. There are a number of better ways for approaching the subject. Suppose, for instance, that you are suffering from arthritis. The pain is not going away and you think a specialist might have another idea:

"You've been giving me very good care and there are no simple solutions for arthritis, but do you think someone who specializes in this problem might have additional suggestions?"

You, the patient, are in charge, and can see anybody you want. Still, the more you include your doctor in your decision making, the better the results are likely to be. If a doctor is struggling with a difficult problem, a second opinion may actually provide some relief. But, just as patients are often afraid to ask for them, doctors hesitate to recommend them. One reason used to be financial and it is becoming so again with managed care. Doctors may not think that you want to spend the money, or your health-care plan may not make allowances for the consultation. Some doctors fear patients will think they are punting the responsibility and end up feeling rejected. Others are afraid patients will think less of them for it, that they're not up to the job. One doctor told me,

"My patients expect that I know everything, so when I suggest getting a second opinion, to them it means that I need help."

If you're afraid of offending your doctor by requesting a second opinion, try asking for a recommendation:

"Do you have someone you would like me to see?"

Even if all your friends have been telling you about a doctor that you should try, remember that popularity doesn't necessarily reflect technical competence and honesty. In many instances, one particular doctor gets a big name in the community and it becomes socially acceptable to go to him, almost like going to the trendiest restaurants that are not always the best. Ask the doctor about this consultant and listen if he has reservations. If you say,

"I heard SoAndSo knows a lot about arthritis. Do you think I should go to him?"

you've made a legitimate request but it may not get you optimal results. It is indeed better than going behind the doctor's back, but there are less threatening ways of making the suggestion:

"Have you heard of Dr. SoAndSo? Do you think he's someone who could give us some help with this?"

And if the doctor responds with, *"I know someone I think is better,"* then it might be a good idea to try his recommendation first.

There is no general formula for effective cooperation with your physician. Each relationship has to be worked out on an individual basis. Find a doctor you can trust and one who is open to negotiation.

It helps to be well informed as long as you don't challenge the doctor. Before asking questions, search your soul as to why you are asking. Is the question relevant to your health problem? Is there something you really want to know or are you asking for another reason? Think about whether you trust the doctor. If there is something that worries or confuses you, try to find a nonabrasive way of asking about it:

"I don't quite understand why you have to do that test, could you please explain it again? I'm really worried."

As a patient, when I have found myself unsure about something, I learned to rephrase the doctor's words when asking a question, *"I remember you said that the reason I . . . ."* Although it's hard, try to reach out and put yourself in the doctor's position. It will make you more sensitive to how you're coming across and what the doctor has to deal with. Although you may think it's the doctor's job to assess and communicate with patients, you are just as important a partner in the communication process. Try not to expect too much—be realistic. Doctors already have unrealistic expectations of themselves, and when you add more to their job, you're setting yourself and the doctor up for failure. Remember that you are there for help, not to impress, win an argument, or come out ahead. You are there to give the information and communicate how you are feeling and what you are concerned about in such a way that the doctor can understand, respond, and help.

WHY DON'T I FOLLOW
MY DOCTOR'S ADVICE?

▼
▼

Do you always do what your doctor tells you? If you do, you're the exception to the rule. Do you have any idea how often people go to the doctor and then don't do anything they were told to do? It may seem surprising how frequently this happens in light of the fact that going to the doctor takes courage and is also inconvenient and expensive. Why, then, do so many patients fail to follow medical advice after taking the trouble to make an appointment, rearrange their schedules, and actually drive somewhere out of the way? Some make appointments and then don't keep them. As many as 40 percent who make appointments because they are sick never show up. Worse yet, 60 percent of patients who are health conscious enough to make appointments for preventive measures—ranging from diet advice to blood pressure checkups—never actually darken the doctor's doorstep.[1] Out of 750 million prescriptions written in the United States and the United Kingdom every year, as many as 520 million are not even filled.[2]

And while you may assume that you are more likely to cooperate if you have to pay for a service, that is not necessarily true.

In my early studies of patient noncompliance at Cornell, most of our physicians simply assumed that noncompliance was the patients' fault, labeled the patients as "uncooperative," and more or less wrote them off. But, as doctors, we were surprised when we discovered that the lack of cooperation we were witnessing could often be explained by our own behavior. The problem was not related to the technical aspects of medical care but, in fact, primarily the result of human aspects. Patients were not happy with the way the doctors had behaved toward them. In questionnaires, they wrote,

> *The doctor didn't listen to me . . . .*
> *The doctor didn't understand me . . . .*
> *The doctor didn't really understand why I came to see her . . . .*

Have you ever felt that way? I hear these same sentiments echoed by patients today, almost half a century later. What I found then is still true today—when patients are not satisfied, they rarely follow their doctors' advice.

I remember an encounter in which a mother brought her toddler in to see one of our doctors, hoping to get medicine for a bad cough that was keeping the whole family awake at night. She expected a strong prescription to stop the cough, but when the doctor examined her little girl, he knew that it would be important for her to continue coughing to bring up mucus. The child had a sinus infection and a postnasal drip, which was causing the coughing. The physician prescribed nose drops, the use of a vaporizer, and an antibiotic. He tried to explain that a medicine strong enough to suppress the cough is bad for growing children, that the cough was serving a purpose, and that such a medicine would relieve only one symptom of the infection, not the cause. Although he thought that the mother was satisfied when she left, we later learned that she had gone over to the pharmacy and bought an over-the-counter cough syrup. She had not followed any of his advice because she had not grasped how it related to her main expectation.

When patients' expectations for a specific treatment are not acknowledged, they typically walk out saying,

"That doctor never did understand what's the matter with me. All I wanted was some cough medicine but he wouldn't give it to me."

Even if a doctor does give a satisfactory explanation of why he or she feels no medication is needed, it won't help unless the patient feels truly understood. The doctor who automatically writes out a prescription achieves a high level of patient satisfaction, but over the long haul it may backfire. A prescription written just to please is based on a dishonest assessment of the situation and is counterproductive. It becomes a collusion between doctor and patient. Moreover, if the prescription does not work, the patient then loses trust.

I know of a patient who developed a cold with all of the typical symptoms—cough, sore throat, congestion. She made an appointment with her doctor with the full intention of getting an antibiotic. When he examined her, he quickly looked at her throat, listened to her chest, and took her blood pressure.

DOCTOR: *Why don't I just write you out a prescription for an antibiotic?*

PATIENT: *Sure, thanks.*

She had gotten what she came for. But she had previously heard that antibiotics work only on either viruses or bacteria and she couldn't remember which. To satisfy her curiosity, she asked him which it was.

DOCTOR: *Oh, of course, antibiotics work for bacteria only.*

He began writing. She began to wonder how he knew which one she had.

PATIENT: *So then I have a bacteria?*

DOCTOR: (Indignantly) *Of course you have a bacterial infection. I wouldn't have given you the antibiotics otherwise.*

When I met this patient, she told me about what had happened and asked me how her doctor knew her cold had been caused by bacteria. I explained that there was no way he could have known without doing a culture. Yet, from experience he knew that, with rare exception, when patients come in with the minor symptoms of a cold, they expect a prescription for antibiotics. He was very busy and did not take the time to explain that antibiotics wouldn't work because he knew what she expected.

Do you think the doctor should prescribe a treatment for everything that's wrong? Many patients expect that there is a treatment for everything. That's one of the reasons why prescribing unnecessary medications is very common. Physicians are on tight time schedules and frequently fear that it will take too long to help patients understand why they are not getting a prescription. If you are adamant and want that prescription no matter what, it will take a doctor who is very patient and sure of himself not to just give in and say,

"Okay, I'll give you an antibiotic for your cold,"

in hopes that you will leave satisfied and tell your friends about him. Patients often insist and push their doctors to the point where they simply give in just to get rid of them. Yielding to the pressure by giving unnecessary medication sometimes seems the simplest way to satisfy. When physicians are accused of prescribing unnecessary drugs, they blame patients:

"Oh, she wouldn't have been satisfied unless I gave it to her."

But patient satisfaction is really not based on whether they get medicines or not, but on whether they think their doctors understood their concerns.

What causes people to either follow or ignore advice? In our studies of large numbers of patient visits in a variety of settings, we found that close to one-half of the patients felt that their main concerns had not been addressed and that their expectations had not been met.[3]

When we first began studying compliance, we learned that you are more likely to follow advice in a setting where you see the same physician over time because it allows you to develop a strong relationship. This continues to be true, but may become more of a problem now that health-care delivery is changing and continuity of care is becoming more difficult to achieve. In fact, our studies showed that the strongest predictor of compliance is the quality of the relationship. It also turns out that some of the myths—such as that educated patients are better at following advice—are untrue. Physicians, for instance, are among the most noncompliant patients in the world! And people assume that patients who are financially well off are more compliant, but that is also untrue.

What is true is that there are certain personality traits associated with good follow-through. Have you ever wondered whether your efforts at controlling your diet, leading a healthy lifestyle, and getting lots of exercise really make a difference? Or do you believe in fate? Patients who have high self-confidence, good self-esteem, and believe that they are the master of their own fate are among those most likely to follow doctor's orders. But, as you might expect, people who are fatalistic and believe that some power outside themselves will determine whether they will live or die are usually less motivated to follow advice.

"When it's my time to go, it's my time to go. Why should I go to the doctor?"

They count on luck, destiny, and fate, and consequently don't believe that taking actions for their health could make a difference.

Do you always do what's good for you? Most physicians are, at heart, missionaries and want to educate patients. They frequently think that if patients have knowledge about their health, they will adopt the appropriate behavior. But it is not just a matter of whether patients understand what their doctors tell them. Doctors frequently say:

"If I could only make him understand, he would do it."

Obviously if the doctor does not explain things clearly and the patient consequently does not understand, it poses a barrier to follow-through. But even if you do comprehend what to do, you may not do it. Socrates, back in the fourth century B.C., embraced the principle,

To know the good is to do the good.

However, Socrates' contemporary, Euripides, in his play *Hippolytus*, has Phaedra show her feminine insight by stating that this is not necessarily so:

We know the good, we apprehend it clearly.
But we can't bring it to achievement. Some are
betrayed by their own laziness, and others value
some pleasure above virtue.

Her words state the problem with great clarity. It seems logical to think that when you go to the doctor, you will cooperate because you are there for your own health. If we are reasonable, why shouldn't that be true? Yet, it's not the way most people behave.

Taking the prescribed treatment will not be high on your priority list if you don't think the illness is serious and if the medication does not seem to be doing anything. What motivates you to follow advice is not what your doctor thinks but, instead, what *you* think. There are many different explanations for why we ignore what we are told. Some people simply forget to take their medicine. Others lose motivation to continue taking medication if they think it has already helped. But, if the drug does not work fast enough, patients will also neglect to take it. And while you might think that patients who must take medications over extended periods of time get used to it and follow through, the opposite is true.

Let's look at a case. A patient's routine skin test comes back positive for tuberculosis. Although she is feeling fine, her physician instructs her to take several daily medications for months. Because she is not feeling sick and the medication does not relieve any symptoms, she does not perceive the gravity of her situation and fails to take the medicine. Not only does she risk developing tuberculosis, she also endangers the community. Whose fault is it? How could it have been prevented? If the patient had insisted by saying, *"Why do I have to do this?"* or if the physician had volunteered an explanation of the medicines' purpose, the situation might have been prevented.

Simple regimens are more likely to be followed than complex ones. It's easier to take a medication once a day than three times a day. Very few patients can actually take a medication faithfully four times a day for a prolonged period of time. Having to take a pill morning, noon, afternoon, and bedtime for more than a day or two is nearly impossible for most of us. One exceptionally motivated patient who had kidney disease and hypertension wore three wrist watches with alarms and set each one for the time when a different medication was due. Unfortunately, most of us are not as dedicated, and physicians don't always think about that when writing out prescriptions.

Another cause of noncompliance are the side effects of medications. This is especially true if you do not know about them beforehand and your doctor does not explain them. Medicines for high blood pressure, for example, may make you feel sleepy. Although you know that if you take your pills, you will be less likely to have a stroke or a heart attack in thirty years, you may end up not taking them because you find yourself falling asleep at work. It becomes a question of priority. An acquaintance of mine who was in an automobile accident and broke her leg was given a prescription for pain by the emergency room physician. When she later had it filled, she noted that the list of side effects included nausea and vomiting. Even though she was in pain, she immediately threw the medication away.

"For me, nothing's worse than being sick to your stomach," she told me, *"and there's no way I'm going to take that chance."* The doctor had never discussed what the possible side effects of the drug were. If he had, he might have reassured her or she might have requested an alternate treatment. In fact, she did not even see the doctor write out the prescription; it was given to her by one of the nurses with the explanation,

"Here, this is for the pain."

Sometimes treatment interferes with daily activities and sometimes patients simply don't like the way it makes them look. Advice that results in changing our appearance, such as recommendations for eyeglasses, hearing aids, or canes, may be unacceptable because of the images these devices conjure up. One of my patients was failing in school and still refused to wear her hearing aid because she was being teased about it. There are people who are so nearsighted that they bump into doors yet still refuse to wear their glasses. People ignore advice to stay out of the sun because they like the way they look with a tan.

This kind of problem can take on dramatic, even life-threatening proportions in certain situations. Years ago I was working with a group of physicians and surgeons who were caring for patients with end-stage kidney disease. Our patients were desperately ill teenagers who had renal failure and had received kidney transplants. Intellectually, all of them understood the grave ramifications of not taking the immuno-suppressive drugs;

they had all been warned that if they did not take them, their kidneys could be rejected or they could even lose their lives.

It never occurred to us that our patients would actually interrupt taking these life-saving medications. But quite a few patients did stop taking their medication, which caused some to have kidney damage and others to actually lose their transplants. We never even suspected that anything was wrong until certain side effects caused by the drugs—weight gain around the face and acne—started to disappear.

These patients did not dare tell us that they had stopped taking the medicines, and for several weeks we had no idea what was actually going on. When we realized what was happening, we were absolutely furious. We felt personally betrayed and it was difficult for some of our team members to continue to empathize with these patients. Kidneys are scarce, transplant surgeries are complex and dangerous, and so much time and money had been invested. The physicians had made tremendous sacrifices for them; they spent hours with patients before and after surgery, lost night after night of sleep, and had maintained their lives throughout dialysis with all of the inherent complications. I heard them say over and over:

"How could you do this to us after all we have done for you?"

One young woman had recently begun junior college, had an active social life, and was very pretty with a slim figure and beautiful long hair. After her transplant, she was on high doses of the medication and experienced the typical side effects—her hair began to change, she developed bad acne, she gained a lot of weight, and her face got round from the cortisone. She told me, *"If I'm going to look like this, I don't want to go back to school, I'd rather be back on dialysis."* A few of the other girls echoed her sentiments. For some of the more vulnerable, the fact that the drugs had caused their appearance to become so bad made the treatment intolerable. Even though we had made a sincere effort to explain the nature and the short duration of the side effects, they told us,

"It's not worth it."

The doctors had the opposite viewpoint. One commented to me,

"When doctors are busy saving lives, it's hard to take a little skin rash or change in appearance sufficiently seriously to empathize with the patient's feelings."

Sometimes there are cultural or religious objections to parts of the treatment. In certain cultures, families refuse to allow their adolescent daughters to have breast or pelvic exams because it taints their value as women. Jehovah's Witnesses strongly believe that they will not go to heaven if they receive blood or blood products. Recently, a young girl was brought to the hospital in need of major surgery, and when her parents read the official consent form, there was a clause stating that it was possible that she could require a blood transfusion during the operation. Her parents refused the operation because they did not want to take that risk, which put their doctors in an ethical bind. As conscientious physicians, they would not undertake a complex operation without the option of giving a blood transfusion. The choices were to try to persuade them to accept the blood transfusion, to let the patient go without urgent surgery, or send them to a facility where someone might be willing to compromise.

Some of our doctors felt that we should try to override the parents' objections and take them to court. This would have placed the doctors in a completely adversarial relationship with the family. Even if that had been their choice, it was not certain that the judge would rule in favor of the medical establishment. In fact, in most cases, judges take the patient's side. And in this case, the young girl herself also expressed strong objections to having a transfusion or any other blood product. When our attempts at persuasion failed, the family went to another facility where the doctors agreed to do the surgery without giving blood. Luckily, all went well.

There are, then, many patient attributes, value systems, and motivational issues that determine whether a particular patient will be able to follow medical advice. How about the other end of the equation? What is it about doctors that might influence a patient's compliance? Do you think that who the physicians are and how they present themselves makes a difference in whether you will follow their advice? Do you prefer your doctor to be older or younger? How do you feel if your physician wears khakis and tennis shoes instead of a formal business suit? Should your doctor wear a white coat?

One of the interns I supervise is from India and he wears a turban. During an appointment, he came out of the examination room and told me that his patient, a six-year-old girl, was being very uncooperative. She wouldn't do anything he asked and screamed when he came near her. I thought right away that he probably looked very different from anyone she had ever seen in real life—with his dark beard and turban he looked like Aladdin or a menacing stranger. I went in and began talking to the little girl. Although she was still teary-eyed and upset, I had no trouble examining her. She had calmed down and behaved appropriately. I asked her father if she always became so upset when visiting the doctor. He replied,

> *"No, but she has never seen anyone who looks like him before and she was scared!"*

While it is not surprising that a six year old would react to the way her doctor looked, adults are much the same. During the sixties, the medical establishment frowned on the young, unconventional physicians who wore their hair long, grew beards, and dressed in blue jeans and sandals. We even had an orthopedist who would not let physicians with beards scrub in the operating room, even if they were willing to cover them up with the bottom flaps of the surgical cap. It wasn't a matter of being worried about hygiene, it was the idea of how it looked to the Chief of Orthopedics.

At that time, a study was conducted to see what kind of attire adolescents preferred their doctors to wear.[4] There were four groups of doctors who wore clothing ranging from formal business suits to jeans and sandals. Everybody thought that the teenagers would respond better to physicians who were more like themselves. As it turned out, even the teenagers placed more trust in the doctors who were more professionally dressed in their white coats, and were more likely to take their advice. In general, patients in many different settings seem to prefer physicians who present themselves in a more businesslike and professional manner.

Negotiating

Physicians and patients often think of medical advice primarily as something that is given and not negotiated. After visiting the doctor, few of us are likely to say,

"The doctor and I discussed whether I could . . . and together we worked out this great idea."

What we usually end up saying is something like:

"My doctor told me that I'd better . . . Stop smoking! Stop drinking! Stop eating! Exercise more! Cut out salt!"

You are given impossible goals that you know you can't follow, which only makes you feel worse.

Some decades ago, a physician who headed a well-known clinic in Boston that specialized in treating diabetes used to conduct lecture tours around the country during which he would discuss four or five of his patients who had never experienced any complications. They had never gone into coma or hypoglycemic shock, and they had normal vision and kidney function. He used these patients as proof of the effectiveness of his treatment. But if questioned about how many patients cooperated fully with the treatment, he had to admit that only 10 percent were actually able to follow his entire regimen. For those it was perfect. And for the 90 percent of patients who couldn't, he did not feel they were his responsibility. Unfortunately, this general attitude is typical of many physicians. They feel that lack of cooperation is entirely the patient's problem.

Some doctors believe they are shortchanging their patients if they don't insist on the absolute best. Would the "uncooperative" diabetic patients have done better if the doctor had been willing to discuss some alternate approaches to managing their diabetes even if it wasn't "perfect"? Suppose you are the doctor. You see a patient who is eating himself to death and weighs 240 pounds. His blood pressure is going up, he is getting no exercise. Your medical training, everything you have learned, tells you,

He's gotta stop eating! Now!

You are a humanistic physician and you desperately want to help. What's your best move? You sit the patient down and say,

"You must start losing weight immediately. I will give you a 1200-calorie diet. At the same time, you have to start to exercise every day, at least for an hour."

If your patient follows your advice, he will definitely lose weight. But will he be able to do it? Most patients know perfectly well that they are overweight and would like to lose weight, but after listening to an admonition that they cannot possibly live up to, they feel ashamed and embarrassed. Left without any practical guidelines, they might actually begin to eat more. One option they have is just not to return to you—this is, in fact, what most people do. If the guidelines aren't realistic and the patient knows she will fail, she gives up before trying. Yet, if doctors acknowledge patients' ambivalence and the dilemma they are facing in making decisions, improvement is more likely.

At one of the clinics of Los Angeles County Hospital we observed a young white female physician examining a dignified older black man. He was extremely thin and seated uncomfortably on the examining table with his clothes off. She began asking him important questions, all the while roughly manipulating his head and neck. And while he struggled to tuck his shirt into his trousers, she interrogated:

DOCTOR: *Who are you living with right now?*

PATIENT: *Well, friends of mine, name of Richards.*

DOCTOR: *Who cooks for you?*

PATIENT: *His wife. He and his wife both cook.*

DOCTOR: *Are you eating three meals a day?*

PATIENT: *Well, sometimes.*

DOCTOR: *Why aren't you eating three meals a day all the time?*

PATIENT: *I just don't have the appetite for it, just can't eat.*

DOCTOR: *Have you always had a poor appetite?*

PATIENT: *Always.*

DOCTOR: *So you never had a good appetite?*

PATIENT: *Never.*

DOCTOR: *Tell you what. Would you make me a promise? Two promises.*

PATIENT: *It all depends.*

DOCTOR: *One is that you will stop smoking. Huh?*

PATIENT: (Laughs) *No!*

DOCTOR: *You won't promise that?*

PATIENT: *No.*

DOCTOR: *Well, will you think about it?*

PATIENT: *I'll think about it, but I won't promise.*

DOCTOR: *And the other thing. Will you start eating three meals a day?*

PATIENT: *I'll think about that too.*

DOCTOR: *You'll have to do better than that, okay? You have to sit down and eat three meals a day. You've lost five pounds. Will you do that for me? Okay?*

The approach this doctor uses to enlist the patient's cooperation is an unfortunate one. Without exploring his life situation or attitudes, she abruptly demands that he change basic habits. A brief interview with him after the visit revealed that not only was his appetite poor, but that he relied on food stamps, which would make it next to impossible for him to follow her suggestions. Like many doctors, she thinks that scaring him about his weight loss will add fuel to his motivation. She attempts to extract promises in a patronizing manner. Demanding a promise of a responsible adult is demeaning and would have stopped most patients in their tracks. Why should he promise her anything? Promises are inappropriate in brand-new relationships. Fortunately, this resourceful old man had the courage to challenge her by simply saying, "*No.*" This caused her to back off a little with: "*You won't promise me that? Well, will you think about it?*" Although he did not acquiesce, he did say that he would think about it. This might have been her next chance to reconsider her approach, but she dropped the ball.

When it comes to altering ingrained habits, almost all patients are ambivalent. Although you may be motivated to actively treat an illness, a urinary tract infection, for instance, you may not be quite as enthusiastic if your doctor asks you to change your eating habits. You may or may not be ready to change. For the most part, doctors do not acknowledge this and simply give instructions. They fail to consider that lifestyle habits develop over time and not without reason. These habits may not be desirable from a health perspective, but they must have been meeting some of the patient's needs. If a couple goes out to dinner and one person orders a big, rich meal, it makes it difficult, if not impossible, for the other to have only a salad. A manager in a stressful job feels she can't get through the day without stepping outside and having a cigarette. Giving that up overnight could be so stressful that it would jeopardize her performance.

In the world of medicine, disease and treatment are everything. Physicians just don't think of the day-to-day worries and lifestyles of their patients. They put life on hold and put the patient's health first; but few patients give their health the highest priority. Doctors so often complain,

> *"My patient will not cooperate!"*

Cooperation, however, is an interactive process. It would be more accurate if they said,

> *"I failed to obtain that patient's cooperation."*

Patients cannot cooperate all by themselves—it takes two. In an ideal world, you would hope a doctor would bridge the gap and see it from the patient's perspective, but in real life it is not that easy.

Experience has shown that telling a patient what to do without first assessing what that person's own ideas are about the treatment, whether or not the patient is even motivated to change, and how ready the patient is to alter a lifestyle, often results in frustration for both patient and physician. But if the physician is empathic with the patient's difficulty in making these changes, the results are likely to be better than when the physician abruptly issues demands. Frustration on both sides can be reduced by negotiating medical advice, especially when it involves lifestyle changes. As a patient, make your physician aware of your situation, your state of mind, and your readiness and motivation to make a change. This will enable your doctor to empathize with your dilemma and give you more realistic advice.

Scare Tactics

When patients do not cooperate, many physicians use scare tactics to motivate them. Every medical interaction is already saturated with fear before the physician deliberately attempts to scare the patient. Have you ever gone in for a visit where you didn't experience the slightest twinge of fear? Patients often expect to be afraid and they often feel they *need* to be that way in order to do what they're supposed to do. And, to a limited degree, that's true. A moderate amount of fear may be a good motivator.[5] But being really scared can have the opposite effect and cause people to deny, withdraw, and get defensive. I, for example, was one of the last people to wear seat belts in a car. I hated the idea of being tied down. In my heart, I always thought it was more dangerous to wear them than not. Then one time when I got into a car with another doctor, she fastened her seat belt and then waited for me to fasten mine.

"Aren't you going to put on your seat belt?" she asked. I quipped that I had had a long life and that I wasn't really afraid of dying in an accident. She thought a moment and then said, *"But you might not die, you might just lose your front teeth!"* I immediately put on my seat belt. She had presented a scenario I could respond to. The fear of my own death was not going to make me change my ways because I simply could not deal with the very idea. But the threat of losing my front teeth was something that I could respond to and take steps to prevent.

Some years ago, our endocrinology department referred a young woman to me because she had been highly noncompliant with her treatment for long-standing diabetes. She was supposed to be on a strict diet, giving herself injections three times a day, and testing her urine and blood as many as five times a day. For the last two years, she had frequently interrupted all aspects of the regimen. In the course of the interview, we had the following exchange.

> PATIENT: *A year, year and a half ago, I stopped taking care of myself because I got sick of them* (the injections). *I would get mad, I would look at the medicine, I would look at the needles, I would throw [them] away.*

> DOCTOR: *Were you afraid when you stopped? Had they told you that bad things might happen to you if you didn't take it?*

PATIENT: *Yeah, they told me about the eyesight about a year ago and they told me that I could die, but that's all they told me.*

DOCTOR: *Did you believe them?*

PATIENT: *A little . . . . I pushed it out of my mind.*

DOCTOR: *You just didn't think about it?*

PATIENT: *Uh huh. I would get my medicine and then I would look at it and then I would start to cry . . . you know . . . and say to myself, "Why do I have to take this?" Then I would throw the insulin in the toilet and throw away the syringe.*

This young woman had been threatened with the most devastating consequences—amputation, blindness, kidney-machine treatments, even death. All these threats were so overwhelming that she reacted by denying and rejecting, and "pushing it out of her mind." Later, during the same interview, we continued our conversation:

DOCTOR: *How about being scared? They say, "If you don't do it, something terrible will happen." Does that work for you?*

PATIENT: *No, because they tell me that they have friends who are twenty years old who have diabetes and who are blind . . . have kidney problems, or they don't have a leg.*

DOCTOR: *They tell you that here at the hospital?*

PATIENT: *Yes.*

DOCTOR: *How does that make you feel?*

PATIENT: *I don't feel nothing . . . .*

Health professionals will go far to frighten patients in the mistaken belief that it will make them cooperate, that it will ultimately be good for them.

When doctors frighten patients, they have an obligation to help them deal with their fears. Doctors should always let you know that they will be there for you and, if possible, they should give you information and a specific plan of action to help reduce your anxiety. If you find yourself becoming afraid, help the doctor shift away from scare tactics by saying:

"I understand it's really very dangerous, but what I need from you now is some help."

The only time when arousing fear can really be justified is when the physician links it with something you can do:

"Insulin-dependent diabetes at your age is a very serious condition, but if you take the insulin regularly and stay on a sensible diet, there's no reason you shouldn't enjoy good health for the rest of your life."

Or,

"Your blood pressure is very high but if we begin to work on your weight, it will most probably come down."

If you are unable to deal with all of the contingencies that the doctor presents, try to negotiate by expressing how you feel:

"I realize you really want me to do this and that's why you're telling me all of the terrible things that could happen if I don't. But at the moment I'm really overwhelmed. I'm scared and I'm not sure I'm going to remember what you're saying."

It may not be until you get home that you sense how frightened you were. You start telling someone what happened and realize how you actually feel. If you find yourself overwhelmed and feeling helpless, your doctor may have been insufficiently aware of your feelings. Either by phone or during your next visit, ask for reassurance and further explanation:

"You mentioned some awful things that might happen to me. How likely is that? You really scared me. How likely is it that I will actually have to go through all that?"

In another dramatic excerpt from my conversation with the diabetic young woman, she sadly told me about her lack of family support. In negotiating problems in compliance, one of the issues doctors need to explore is what type of support the patient may be able to enlist in following a difficult treatment regimen. Social support is important from an emotional point of view so that you don't feel alone and have someone to turn to. This is especially true at times of stress and illness. It's very hard to carry out a complex treatment regimen alone, and so I asked the young woman if her family took an interest in her illness:

> PATIENT: *No. . . . they tease me a lot. They go out and buy cakes and cookies and all that.*
>
> DOCTOR: *Do you talk to them about that?*
>
> PATIENT: *No because . . . ummm they're like . . . I don't talk to my father and they do . . . and I call my dad names, you know . . . . I call him a name and they will start saying "Don't call him that, he's your dad." I call him this because he doesn't care and he doesn't ask for me and when I am in the hospital he hardly comes or he doesn't even come and visit me.*

Her sisters were undermining her diet. She and her father had a bad relationship and he took no interest in her illness or hospitalization. How could she possibly have carried out the daily instructions of three insulin shots plus five urine and blood tests? In some of the studies of patient cooperation with treatment regimens, one of the factors that was found to be crucial was not only family support but also communication about the illness. If no one is willing to talk about it, if the treatment is not discussed, it is harder for the patient to deal with it. In yet another incident, when the young woman did not give herself the insulin and hid the syringe, her mother discovered what she had done:

> PATIENT: *One day my mom found out. I was going to "put on" my insulin that day but I didn't want to do it at that time. I was going to save it and in the rest room there is a thing up there and I climbed up there and hid it and I guess my mom was cleaning and she found out. And when I came back she was mad at me . . . she just stared at me and didn't tell me nothing . . . but she told my dad.*

There was a deplorable lack of communication in this family. Her mother made no attempt to sit down and talk things over. Instead, she reported her daughter's "bad behavior" to her father, her enemy. If the mother could have discussed the treatment with her daughter, perhaps she could have helped. Even if there is just one person who shows interest—perhaps a good friend—patients are much more likely to comply.

It is often difficult for doctors to contemplate the fact that their advice might not work or that a particular patient might not follow through. An observation we made many times in our study of doctor–patient encounters is that doctors do not consider the possibility that patients fail to take their medicines. Patients, in response, do not dare bring it up. This not only causes a rift in the doctor–patient relationship but also reduces the likelihood of open communication in the future.

A typical subject in our study was a mother who had been bringing her son to our clinic for treatment of epilepsy. When we interviewed her after an appointment and asked if her son was able to take the medication and whether she gave it the way the doctor prescribed, she told us, *"No, he was so sleepy in school, he couldn't do the work so I cut it in half. . . . I took away the morning dose so he would stay awake."* In the meantime, she had told the doctor that her son had had several seizures, but left out the part about how she had not been giving the full dose. The doctor then doubled the dose without knowing that she was keeping him in the dark about how much his patient was actually taking.

Some physicians feel it's their job to give it to you straight and then leave everything else up to you. They see their responsibility as making a diagnosis, prescribing the right medicine, and not worrying about whether you actually take it. Some are willing to negotiate and make you a part of the decision making. Although some patients are able to handle the advice from perfectionist doctors who simply tell you what to do, others cannot. It's a different mind-set and it is something to consider in selecting your physician. Your quality of life while you are taking the medication is a lot more important to you than it is to your doctor. What approach works the best for you? It's up to you to decide on your priorities and let your doctor know what you want and need.

What Can You Do?

In discussing treatment, think about the issues that are most important to you. Do you have questions to ask? When you are given a prescription, don't just say thank you and walk out of the office knowing that you can't follow it. Don't pretend to be able to do something you know you can't. Be honest about your concerns and negotiate something that you will be able to handle. If you have doubts, don't hesitate to say,

> *"I don't think I can remember to take this four times a day."*

Then ask for help in solving the problem:

> *"Is there some other medication that doesn't require that I take it as often? Isn't there some way you could give me something different so I could take it before I leave home and then not until I get home at night?"*

Never feel foolish if you have to ask your doctor more than once about what a medication does. Although your pharmacist can help with general knowledge about your medication, possible side effects, and how you are to take it, only your doctor knows you. And it is your doctor who is best suited to give you individualized advice about the aim of the treatment and what it should do for you.

You have a right to negotiate your treatment and an obligation to let your doctor know to what extent you feel it is something you can do. If you don't like to take medicines unless they are absolutely necessary, say so. If you haven't been taking the medicine, be sure to speak up. There is no way physicians can help if they think you are taking medications when you are not, or not taking them as instructed. There are items you can ask for. You may want written instructions, a phone call follow-up, further reading, and other memory aids such as pill boxes with compartments for every day of the week, special calendars, or refrigerator notes.

It is important to inquire how the treatment relates to your illness so that you understand the importance of taking the medication as instructed. I had a patient whose mother put penicillin drops in her ear that were meant to be swallowed. I had given very specific instructions that the drops were to be taken by mouth. But she didn't understand how drops swallowed would do the ear any good. She was too embarrassed to ask me to repeat the explanation and I had no idea that she had not understood.

Make it clear that you don't necessarily expect a prescription but that you do want the doctor to understand how sick you feel and how worried you are. When physicians do not hand out prescriptions, we patients may feel as if our sickness and worry have not been acknowledged. It is our responsibility to make ourselves heard. When you've got a streaming nose, a pounding headache, and can't swallow because of a sore throat, if your doctor says, *"Oh, you've just got a cold and there is no need for an antibiotic,"* you very well may feel invalidated. You *feel* as if you need an antibiotic or some strong prescribed drug that will alleviate your symptoms. Make sure your doctor has gotten your message by calmly saying,

> *"I don't necessarily expect medicine but I do want you to know how bad I feel in case it is something more serious."*

If you don't believe your doctor understands how sick you are, stop a moment and briefly voice your main concern:

> *"You know, I have not slept through a whole night for two weeks. I am worried that this might be developing into something more serious."*

Patients worry when symptoms persist for a long time. If that's the way you feel, say:

> *"Do you realize how long I've had this? It has been three weeks and I am very concerned."*

Do We Really Need That Prescription?

No matter how minor the problem, we almost always expect *something*—a prescription, a test, an MRI. And when we don't get it, we feel as if we are getting second-class service. In a civilization where technical services, tests, and medications are constantly being huckstered, we are following the lead by demanding tests and medications that we may not need. Products are almost literally pushed down our throats—through ads on TV and in magazines. There is so much out there that we fail to discriminate between what's important and what's not. And because we now expect so much, we push our doctors to prescribe. And doctors respond by doing so promiscuously. Physicians know that meeting patients' short-term expectations will satisfy them but they have, in effect, created a Frankenstein monster that has gone on the rampage. In the not too distant past, a doctor would listen to your heart and tell you that it sounded good. Nowadays the sophisticated patient says, *"Well, aren't you going to do an electrocardiogram?"* And patients with minor ailments ranging from athletic injuries to migraine headaches commonly ask for MRIs and CT scans.

Nowadays, patients go to their doctors long before they would have in past decades. Even though many of the illnesses we consult doctors about have no real cures or effective treatments, we have become more and more doctor dependent. This is, in part, due to the fact that we are all faced with a seemingly endless list of experts—from preventive medicine specialists who tell us how to avoid strokes and heart attacks to cosmetic surgeons who keep us young and beautiful to sports physicians who help us recover from our "healthy" lifestyle.

Because we get so much advice from so many different directions, we tend to do less of what we are asked. Yet, paradoxically, we are the ones asking for it. The more we feel that every time we sneeze we need somebody to tell us what to do, the less we trust ourselves and the more helpless we become. As affluent as we are, surrounded by entrepreneurs and endless information, we have developed a set of expectations that rightly or wrongly leads to more prescriptions and advice than is perhaps desirable. We have lost confidence in our own wisdom and the wisdom of the body. We have become excessively dependent on a series of experts who are not always in agreement with one another but continue to bombard us, making us feel uncomfortable with our own behavior. We have developed a mind-set in which there is a technical solution for every problem. This leads us to have a set of expectations that sends us to the doctor knowing that he or she will give us something to "fix" the problem.

Patients typically leave the doctor's office asking,

"What about a prescription?"
"Isn't there <u>something</u> I should take?"
"Aren't you going to do any tests?"
"You mean you aren't you going to give me a shot of penicillin?"

As new technologies have been introduced, patients have incorporated them into their expectations. Unfortunately, there are doctors who prescribe antibiotics for viral infections for which they are not likely to be much help. We are now learning that, in the long run, this practice can cause harm. When antibiotics are used too much, our systems can, in effect, develop defenses that render them useless later when we might really need them.

We have become farther and farther removed from what our own bodies and intellect can do, and we need to restore our own trust in finding solutions. It is important to have confidence in our ability to control events, to deal with stress, to have some sense of our own well-being. We are losing confidence that our bodies can heal on their own. Young physicians are always amazed when I remind them that patients did get over infectious diseases before we had antibiotics. Of course, there are many times when we do need medicines, but it is important to remember that we have our own inner resources.

Patients often look at medical advice and being cured of an illness as a process that the doctor does *to* the patient. We have very different roles and the doctors are almost always thought of as the active participants. Yet all research shows that the more patient centered the encounter and the more active the patient, the better the outcome.[6] Patients who are self-reliant, well informed, and highly motivated can help themselves. We are the ones ultimately responsible for changes and improvements in our health. We have the power to influence our relationships with members of the health-care team. Physicians can change treatments and help us better understand our symptoms so that we can take better care of ourselves. But your doctor's worth is not only in knowing the very best drug in the world for your illness, but in working with you to find a way to help you get well.

WHERE IS THE TRUTH?

Secrets and Lies in the Doctor–Patient Relationship

How much information do you think your doctor should give you? One sophisticated patient volunteered, *"I want my doctor to tell me exactly what he would tell a colleague. So, if another doctor asks him about my condition, I want to hear what he says."*

Is that the way you feel? Do you want technical details? If your doctor chooses one treatment, do you want to know all about other possible treatments? The last time you left your doctor's office, did you wonder whether there were things he wasn't telling you? Did you expect your doctor to share all of the information she has about your condition during that particular visit?

A patient of mine said,

> *"My husband and I are very conscientious people, we're very detail oriented. We want as much information as they can give us. Swamp*

me with it. I don't care, I'll go home, I'll sort it out, I'll come back with my questions.

"We need a guess, something so we can sleep at night, just something. We won't hold you to it, just give us a ballpark estimate or your best opinion . . . . This is the way we need to function. Maybe other people don't want to know those things. I need to be told the blunt truth. I mean, give me the worst case and then I'll back up from there."

In contrast, another patient's husband, who had been in a similar situation, said,

"If they [think we] need an operation, we just sign; if they [think we] need medication we say okay. I do not feel that I know enough about anything to question them."

Some patients are very precise and want all the information they can get, from signs and symptoms to numbers and probabilities. Others are exactly the opposite. The tradition in medicine has been not to tell the truth to patients and their families. But the philosophy of not sharing information in medical practice has changed drastically over time. While you may wonder now whether your doctor has withheld important information, you could almost be sure that he would have five decades ago.

There are illustrations throughout history of physicians' conviction that patients were best left uninformed. Hippocrates recommended:

" . . . concealing most things from the patient while you are attending to him . . . revealing nothing of the patient's future or present condition."[1]

According to Oliver Wendell Holmes in an 1871 graduation speech to a medical school class,

"Your patient has no more right to all the truth you know than he has to all the medicine in your saddlebags . . . . He should get only just so much as is good for him . . . . Some shrewd old physicians have a few phrases always on hand for patients who insist on knowing the pathology of their complaints without the slightest capacity of understanding

the scientific explanation. I have known the term 'spinal irritation' to serve well on such occasions."[2]

Eric Cassell, a prominent physician, tells a story that occurred in the 1930s when his own grandmother visited a specialist about a melanoma on her face:

"During the course of the visit when she asked him a question, he slapped her face, saying, 'I'll ask the questions here. I'll do the talking.'"[3]

Cassell comments: *"Can you imagine such an event occurring today? Melanomas may not have changed much in the last fifty years, but the profession of medicine has."*

In the course of my own career, I have experienced drastic changes. As late as the mid-1980s when I was invited to a symposium for surgeons and radiologists at Ville Juif, the main cancer center in the city of Paris, the audience was astounded when I mentioned that, in America, we tell the truth to patients who have cancer or other life-threatening illnesses.

We used to write prescriptions in Latin because we thought the power of the doctor was greater if the patient did not know too much about the medication. When we began translating prescriptions into English in the 1960s, I realized that we were demystifying medicine in a way similar to the way religion was demystified during the Reformation four centuries ago. Until the sixteenth century, religious services were conducted in Latin and the parishioners could not understand much of what was said. So just as the early clergy exercised a great deal of power, physicians today have increased power when they withhold information from their patients.

But in the last few decades, medicine has begun to go through a transformation. Nowadays, we expect our physicians to thoroughly explain each medication they recommend. There are package inserts in medicines that give warnings, and explain side effects, and we have pharmacists to answer our questions about prescribed medications. Bookstores now have shelves of health books, including medical encyclopedias, specialized books about diseases and treatments, and tomes the size of big city telephone directories containing detailed information on just about every drug on the market. Television programs and documentaries show us real-life footage of the latest surgical techniques, and most university medical school libraries are open to the public. Anyone with a PC has access to the World Wide Web. In fact, just about all the information your doctor has is also available to you. And there is speculation now that, as technology advances, a lot more information will be directly available to patients; it may, at times, even take the place of consulting doctors. An example is the poison control centers that have, until recently, been used primarily by physicians. It used to be that when a patient would call a hospital about a child's having taken something toxic, a doctor would call the poison center, find out what to do, and advise the patient. Now patients are often given the poison center's number so that they can call and get the antidote on their own, thus eliminating the physician from the transaction of information. The physician is no longer the only interpreter of medical knowledge.

The Pros and Cons of Sharing Information

So we are trying to demystify medicine. But have we thrown the baby out with the bathwater? Have we diminished our capacity to be helpful to patients? There is no question that doctors have the power to help partly because of the profession's mystique. There's something about having a doctor give you a medicine that goes beyond the exact chemistry of the particular drug. Our doctors have medical expertise and we trust that they know what's best. I love the story one of my colleagues told me about his son. When he arrived home from work one evening, his six-year-old son Mark told him that he had a headache. When doctors finally get home after a long day of seeing sick patients and are told that there is a minor health problem in the family, they are notoriously disinterested: *"Oh, I've been seeing patients all day who are really sick!"* So when Mark complained, his father said, *"Why don't you go and take an aspirin?"* His son lingered and finally asked, *"Aren't you going to give it to me?"* Being given a medicine by a doctor is different from simply taking it ourselves.

A large part of the therapeutic effect of any medication or treatment is the result of the relationship between the doctor and the patient as well as the patient's awareness that he is doing something about the illness. It is well known that patients who take placebos (sugar pills) often do get better more quickly than those who take nothing even though they do not know whether they are receiving the active drug or the placebo in the trial. How could it be that a patient taking a sugar pill will often improve dramatically? The most probable explanation is that the attitude of placebo takers is more positive. They feel they are doing something about their illness. Patients' attitudes can make a difference. In one study, patients with breast cancer who regularly attended support group meetings did better and survived longer than those who did not.[4] In another study, patients with leukemia and related blood cancers were randomized into three groups.[5] One group received extra education that emphasized patients' responsibility for taking an active role in their treatment. Another group received psychosocial support of a very patient-centered type, including visits to the patients' homes. The third group was a control and did not receive either extra education or psychosocial support. There was a significant improvement in the first two groups, including better compliance with medications and prolonged survival time—as long as one year when compared to the control group. No doubt, people who are motivated to do something about their diseases actually do get better.

This raises a question. Who is more effective? Doctors who hold *no* information back from their patients? Or those who withhold information so that they can help their patients have more positive attitudes? What about doctors who give placebos to their patients for symptom relief? To achieve the placebo effect, they cannot be honest with their patients. The old philosophy was that the truth was too upsetting for seriously ill patients and would take away hope. But physicians are now beginning to believe that to be of help, it is best to allow patients to retain their autonomy and deal with the truth in positive ways. This gives us the option of entering into a whole new style of relationship with our doctors—a partnership.

Would you like to think of your doctor more as being a partner in solving your health problems, or would you rather simply trust your doctor to help you? Medical practice and the patient community are leaning in the direction of advocating the partnership relationship between physician and patient. But will our physicians be able to assist us as effectively in that setting? Placebos do work for some patients. But they are dishonest. No answer applies to all doctors, all patients, or all medical encounters. In an all-day seminar devoted to the subject of patient trust, several health professionals in the audience were a bit skeptical about the concept of placing too much trust in your physician. So often, the word "trust" is used in suspicious circumstances. Used car salesmen say, *"Trust me!"* That really means,

"Don't ask any questions, don't do any comparison shopping; trust me to do what's best for you."

So trust is a loaded word. A couple of physicians in the audience even became angry at the speaker. One said,

"Trust is not a desirable thing! It's a blind trust, it means the patient cannot negotiate with the doctor."

On the one hand, a certain amount of paternalism may be therapeutically effective, while on the other, patients should not trust physicians to the extent that they do not ask the appropriate questions. What level of trust is best? All too often, "trust" is blind trust. Most children, for instance, trust their parents and do not question what their parents do for them. By definition, the parent–child relationship is paternalistic. How much of that is helpful to patients in the doctor–patient relationship? Should we trust our doctors to always tell us the truth, to always do what is best? How much do we need to question their decisions? The general trend is toward allowing patients more and more autonomy in making decisions. Although patient autonomy must be respected, it is noteworthy that a significant number of patients express the need for more help and direction.[6] This is especially true when they must make major health decisions.

Is Your Doctor Always Truthful?

It's always a big question as to whom a doctor is protecting when he or she withholds information. Do you think your doctor has ever been less than truthful with you? The same patient who admonished me to "swamp" her with the truth, also said,

"A lot of doctors, we have found, will not make projections at all, or they feel that as patients maybe you're just not able to deal with all the information."

When I asked her if she thought doctors withhold information to protect patients, she answered,

"Partly, I think they're protecting us, but mostly I think they are protecting themselves."

Ideally, patients have a right to be told the truth, and the whole truth, as the doctor sees it. But that may not be the truth either. As Pontius Pilate said, *"What is truth?"*

One of the caveats about telling the truth is that no one really knows the whole truth about every disease or every patient. I learned this lesson dramatically a few years ago when one of my patients brought her baby in to see me. The baby had kidney failure starting early in her first year; usually such children do not grow up to be mentally normal because a condition known as uremia affects the developing brain. Because I was the child's physician, I felt that I owed the mother the "truth." She should know what the kidney experts had told me—that her child would not develop normally. When I told her, she was devastated and left the office in tears. But as things turned out, the medical, scientific "truth" about uremia and the developing brain was not the truth for this child. She grew up completely normal! The mother went through a great deal of unnecessary suffering during the first few years of her child's life and her trust in me was undermined. No matter how many times I tried to explain why I had given her the information, she still deeply resented me. It became her mission in life to prove how wrong I had been. Every year when she came in for checkups, she triumphantly dragged her daughter into the office to show her off: *"Look!"* she'd say, *"she's in second grade, getting all A's."*

As you can see, even telling patients "the truth" has a component of uncertainty that makes it difficult for both sides. As a doctor, all I can do is give my experience. If I am trying to help a patient make a decision and I feel pretty strongly that treatment "A" is a good choice and treatment "B" is not as good, am I actually helping my patient by giving the absolute truth, including my uncertainty?

A patient, Yvonne, recently fell down and severely twisted her ankle while doing routine household chores. When she went to an orthopedist, he told her that she had two options—to have surgery to repair the torn ligaments, which would mean she would wear a cast for six weeks, or to simply wear an ankle brace for three weeks, which would immobilize her foot and allow the wound to repair itself. He told Yvonne that she would probably be able to do "most of the things" she normally did if she elected not to have the surgery. She asked him what he meant by "most of the things" because she is active and loves to run, bike, and scuba dive. He explained that he was fairly sure she would be able to participate in these activities, but that other sports involving ankle twisting, such as skiing, would not be advisable. He also told her that there was no guarantee that surgery would fix the problem 100 percent. Yvonne had one week to make up her mind—after that it would be too late to repair the damage surgically.

This sent her into a quandary. Both alternatives had drawbacks. He had given her his experience and also his uncertainty. Faced with two viable options and wanting "the truth" from him, she asked him what he would do if he were in the same situation. He answered by telling her that he had suffered a similar injury and had elected not to have surgery. But was her injury exactly like his and would her body heal in the exact same way his did? No one could possibly know. When she further pressed him, he said that if he were to use percentages, he was 40 percent in favor of doing the surgery, and 60 percent against. Yvonne found herself confused even more because the numbers were too close. She told me, *"My doctor is just a little bit more against doing the surgery than he is for doing it. That means that there are still quite a few positive points in favor of it. What should I do?"* Her doctor had given her all the "truth" he could by including relative percentages, yet they only further confused her.

Would you want your doctor to give you percentages? Some patients find percentages helpful; others are completely baffled by them. My patient who practically begged to be inundated with information most definitely wanted percentages:

"Just give us a ballpark estimate or your best opinion."

But another patient's husband wanted nothing to do with such information:

"We just had complete faith in them [the doctors]; whatever they said . . . ."

Percentages can be misleading. Percentages had predicted that my patient with kidney failure would be severely brain damaged. But for that one particular case, the percentages couldn't have been less applicable. If you are in the 1 percent who do make it, then it is probably not helpful for you to think too much about the fact that 99 percent do not. Or, conversely, if you are in the 1 percent who don't make it, then you don't care about the other 99 percent who do. One unfortunate patient told me:

> *"When I signed the informed consent before I had cataract surgery, the percentage listed for retinal detachment following the surgery was minuscule, only 3 percent. But that percentage turned out to be devastating for me because I ended up being one of the few unlucky ones. Then the next time I had cataract surgery on my other eye, I was petrified because that tiny 3 percent now seemed gigantic to me and, as it turned out, I again was one of the unlucky ones."*

The mother of a premature baby, Mrs. W., was uneasy asking questions because she felt that the doctors did not want to answer her. Because she is Asian and not completely comfortable with the English language, she had not been able to fully understand previous statements from the doctor at the hospital. Desperate to get information on the likelihood of her baby's survival, she finally confronted another physician whom she trusted and asked for her honest opinion. She specifically requested percentages and was told that there was an 80 percent mortality for such babies. When I interviewed Mrs. W. and inquired why she hadn't asked the doctors at the hospital, she told me:

MRS. W.: *Ah, I didn't give to them any questions. Not any questions, not many questions. Because most people, they don't want to answer, exactly, you know.*

DR. KORSCH: *Do you think if you ask, people don't like it? Do you feel they will think you don't trust them?*

MRS. W.: *No. I think they like to talk, but they don't want to have responsibility of what they're talking.*

DR. KORSCH: *So you figure you had better not ask?*

MRS. W.: *Yes. But I ask my own doctor and what I say to her is—"I'm asking to you personally."*

Here she volunteers that, in her uncertainty, she had returned to her own doctor to ask her question.

> DR. KORSCH: *You asked her "What do you think?"*
>
> MRS. W.: *I ask her how percentage she thinks my child can survive.*

What she wanted to know was what percentage chance her child had of surviving.

> DR. KORSCH: *And what did the doctor say?*
>
> MRS. W.: *That she has an open mind, 80 percent (chance that my baby will die) against the 20 percent chance of the survival. She talked to me surely, that she doesn't care, but ah his, ah, you know—*

Here she means that the doctor was not afraid to take the responsibility of giving an answer even though the doctor was not absolutely certain that she was right.

> DR. KORSCH: *She was not worried about protecting herself?*
>
> MRS. W.: *Ya. Ya. She just open mind, and I'm so happy. I'm so glad about that.*

Eighty percent chance of mortality sounds terrible to most people, but instead of being depressed at the figure, Mrs. W. told me that she instead felt a surge of life. A 20 percent survival rate offered hope.

Do You Want the Truth?

The ambitious young doctors with whom I work have the belief that the best thing to do is tell all they know right away to every patient. The accepted standard, after all, is for doctors to tell the truth. However, the information a doctor gives a patient should be tempered by who the patient is and what he or she is ready to hear. Put yourself in a patient's mind-set. What if you were seriously ill and had only a 20 percent chance of surviving? Would you want to be given that figure? Would it give you hope or dash all your hope? Truth telling takes good judgment and a lot of skill.

I recently had a troubling encounter with a young physician. It was late in the afternoon in our group practice when a mother and her child, who had Down's syndrome, came in for their appointment. Their regular physician was not there that day and so they saw another doctor, whom I'll call Dr. Morris. The mother spoke only Spanish and this doctor had to struggle with the language barrier. On top of that, early in the interview Dr. Morris discovered that she had failed to do what the physician on her previous visit had advised. Visibly upset and very worried, he came to me and told me how the mother had not followed up on any referrals, hadn't done any of the exercises with her baby, and had absolutely no understanding of her child's condition or prognosis. Then he proudly told me that he had now fully informed and educated this mother about Down's syndrome and how it would affect her child.

> *"You know, nobody ever told her what was <u>really wrong</u> with her child and she's been in our clinic five or six times! She doesn't know what Down's syndrome means, how these children never reach normal intelligence, that they may be dependent the rest of their lives, they may never go to a regular school. The total picture of Down's syndrome."*

I reminded him that the other physician may have told her probably more than once, but that patients only hear what they want to hear or what they can deal with. This may have been too much for her and she may not have been able to accept it.

He continued:

> *"But she didn't really know how bad it is, so I told her. She had to understand and now she's crying."*

Nevertheless, he was satisfied that he had done a good job. Yet, he had not only informed her, he had overwhelmed the mother with all that information. And so, at five o'clock that afternoon, she was pushed into facing all the present and future ramifications of having a child with Down's syndrome. When I went into the examination room, she was still in tears, very angry, and wasn't ready to hear anything more. I tried to calm her down, but by that time she was completely unable to listen or respond.

Was the physician right to overwhelm the mother that afternoon with the truth? Was she ready to hear it? Had she been told before? I believe that this doctor had picked the wrong time to give the mother "the truth," and, on top of that, he had never seen her before and made the assumption that she had never been told. He became indignant with me when I spoke with him about timing and dosage of information. He felt that for the doctor to decide how much "truth" a patient is ready for and allowed to know is patronizing and disrespectful of the patient's autonomy. I asked him if he felt that he had really done a good thing that day. Despite the mother's upset, he still felt he had. He later wrote me a two-page letter about the situation and informed me that he felt I was too old-fashioned and paternalistic in my approach and that it was he who truly respected patient autonomy.

If you had been the mother, would you have wanted this doctor to give you the "truth" the way he did? Certainly, one of the current tenets in medicine is that doctors must respect the patient's right to autonomy. Another is that patients should not be deceived by their doctors. Those are two of the most important principles in medical ethics today and they are interrelated. After all, how could you make an autonomous decision about your health or be a true partner in the relationship if your doctor is not telling you everything? Yet doctors are also taught the traditional Latin admonition: *Primum non nocere,* which means "above all, do no harm." And it is possible for doctors to actually do harm by telling the truth. Most of us are aware that patients sometimes sue doctors for not giving them enough information. In rare instances there have been cases in which doctors are sued for presenting the truth in a brutal and unwise way at the wrong time which causes something bad to happen. The ethical principle of "doing no harm" may in fact compete and even conflict with respecting patient autonomy and not deceiving.

Suppose, for instance, that Yvonne with her sprained ankle left the orthopedist's office completely distraught at the idea that what had seemed like a "simple" twisted ankle might now require a rather complex surgery. As she drives home, trying to make what was really an impossible decision, she runs into another car and injures herself as well as the other driver. Now, was her doctor really doing her "no harm" by putting her in a quandary over whether to opt for surgery? He certainly did give her the truth as he knew it, but that truth included his uncertainty. Would she have been better off if he had simply instructed her to wear a leg brace without even bringing up the idea of surgery? But still, if he had done that, he would have been withholding relevant information.

Many contextual variables influence the sharing of information. Among them—who the patient is, who the doctor is, the condition that they are discussing, the time frame of the illness, the patient's need for privacy, the patient's expectations, the complexity of the condition, implications of the illness, and the nature of the patient–physician interaction. Is the surgeon stopping in the hall to speak with the family? Is the surgeon sitting down at the bedside the day following surgery to explain what happened? Are patient and physician conferring during an office visit? Are they talking over the phone? And, is the information that the doctor relays going to affect any action? There are many important considerations.

In a recent lecture by noted oncologist Dr. Alexandra Levine given to her first-year students at the University of Southern California's School of Medicine, she told the story of an elderly lady who had come to her for a second opinion. Her family, who was very concerned and involved in her health care, actually requested that she not be told the truth about her diagnosis. Dr. Levine's new patient was an eighty-six-year-old grandmother who spoke only Spanish, and had been diagnosed to have a malignant lymphoma. Dr. Levine did not believe that her patient would die from the lymphoma; in fact, she was optimistic that she could live for another ten years with the disease. But the patient's very large family (eight children) was petrified by the mere thought of cancer. Before the visit, the family members had gotten together and decided that they would not tell their grandmother what was wrong because they thought that, if she knew, she would be too frightened.

When the time arrived for the appointment, the grandmother came in with one of her daughters who could speak English and had been appointed the spokesperson for the family. The daughter immediately pulled Dr. Levine aside to explain the family's plan of action—the patient was not to be told what she had. Dr. Levine then asked the daughter to talk to the family and try to convince them to agree to tell the grandmother. She would phone the daughter later that afternoon. The daughter agreed to the plan. To make a long story short, the family finally agreed that the grandmother could be informed during her next appointment. The next week when the grandmother arrived, Dr. Levine explained that she had a type of cancer called lymphoma, that she didn't think that it would require drastic treatment, and that she would be the one who took care of her. The grandmother got up from her chair, gave her a big hug, and cried, *"Gracias, gracias mi doctora!"*

She had known it was cancer for some time, but had thought it was much worse than it really was. After all, she was the one who had found a big lump and had taken it on herself to have it biopsied and had even undergone a CT scan and bone marrow tests. Her fears about what was happening inside her were far worse than reality. What the family was doing by keeping the truth from her was, in a sense, pushing her away, making her always alone, never able to say to anyone: *I'm really scared about this, what's going to happen to me?*

When something is wrong, most of us have a tremendous need to share our worries and concerns with our doctors. We may not feel comfortable discussing our problem with anyone else, even close friends or family members. And even if we are able to discuss our problems with acquaintances, the burden is still quite a bit less when we are able to share our thoughts with the one person who knows the most about our health. When doctors withhold information, they distance themselves from their patients and their needs. The patient then carries the burden in isolation. One of the worst experiences for any of us is to be isolated, and being isolated with fear is even worse. Imagine having a health problem, being surrounded by family, friends, and even doctors, and being afraid to tell anyone your thoughts!

The Power of Information

If you knew something about a person that constituted a serious threat to their health yet you were not supposed to tell them, what would you do? There really is no right answer. When a doctor knows something critical about a patient and decides not to tell, then the doctor shoulders quite a heavy burden.

Most of us have been in situations where we know something about an acquaintance, but feel it is not our business to speak up. I've had experiences when I've visited friends and heard something mentioned in passing that really worried me. In one instance, I was at a gathering and noticed that the child of a friend was behaving in a way that suggested early autism. The toddler's parents told me that he was very well behaved, enjoyed playing by himself most of the time and wasn't really interested in other people, that he loved to sit on top of the old-fashioned hi-fi stereo console because he could then watch the records turn, and was fascinated with certain kinds of music. I stood there listening to their description thinking, *Oh no, this may be really abnormal, but it's not bothering the parents and I'm not their doctor.*

While I had been invited there as a friend, not a doctor, I still had quite a bit of knowledge about autistic children that the parents did not. I left the party tremendously worried, yet I did not feel that it was my place to tell the parents what I thought and so the burden of that knowledge remained with me.

Another story Dr. Alexandra Levine told during her lecture involved hope. Her students were impressed to hear this highly regarded specialist relate such a heartfelt story. They did not realize that a technological expert would care so much about patients' feelings.

She tells the story of a patient, a woman in her thirties, whom she had known as a medical student. The patient was outwardly well, physically fit, and had been admitted to the hospital after doctors had discovered a nodule on a chest X ray. This was quite a few years ago, before CT scans, and so the woman was put through a battery of tests that took about a week and turned up nothing. During the week that the young woman was in the hospital, Alexandra, the other students, and the nursing staff got to know her quite well. She was described as "a real dynamo, totally energetic, and outgoing." She became the extra nurse on the ward, ran errands up and down the hospital's fourteen floors, and, by the end of the week, had been unofficially accepted as a member of the nursing team. Her doctors decided to do an exploratory surgery, an "open thoracotomy," to diagnose what had caused the spot on the X ray. They discovered that she had squamous cell carcinoma of the lung, which had already spread widely and could not be surgically removed. The operation was terminated and she was sewn back up again.

The next day, when Alexandra went on rounds with a group of doctors, students, interns, and residents, they went up to the surgical floor and visited the patient's room. The surgeon who had performed the operation leaned over her bed and said,

"Well, it's cancer. We opened and closed. Nothing we can do."

The patient, looking up at him, said,

"Opened and closed?"

She didn't understand what that meant. He again said,

"Yes, we opened and closed."

She repeated it.

"Opened and closed?"

She finally began to get the message, and when the surgeon finally said, *"Anything else?"* the woman shook her head and the rounds group left. Alexandra describes how she stayed behind to try to talk with her and then came back later in the day. *"She had lost her perkiness. It had been easy to talk to her before. Now it was hard. Now I didn't even know what words to use. I was too young to understand what was happening and what I needed to do."*

When Alexandra returned for work the next morning, she was told that the patient had died during the night. It was an unexpected death and, at the autopsy, no specific cause could be determined. Her cancer was in its early stages.

> *"I never understood the case," Alexandra said, "but I believe in my soul that the surgeon's words took away her lifetime. I think what he took away was hope . . . any possibility that there was anything that could be done."*

In my teaching, I emphasize that the kind of information patients are given will make a difference in their attitude about illness, their treatment, and their overall health in general. And that doctors should be aware of the extent to which they are meeting their own needs by giving certain information and to what extent they believe they are helping their patients. In my practice, I make sure that patients know I am always open for questions. I am ready to tell them anything they want to know to the best of my knowledge. And if, for instance, my patient isn't ready for as much as I think is needed, in order to get the best results, I will insist, even at the risk of upsetting the patient. But, on the other hand, if the information isn't that urgent, I try to create a better occasion at a later time to relay what I believe the patient needs to know.

What Is Truth?

In medicine, truth is something we desire but rarely acquire. Medicine is an imperfect art and nothing is certain. If I see a patient with a certain kind of tumor, I might say, on the basis of my experience, that the tumor should be removed within the week. But that patient could be the one case that is different. No one really knows the whole truth. Just think of all those years when women with breast cancer had radical surgery and had their entire breasts removed. Hundreds of thousands of women experienced this mutilation, which was both physically and psychologically traumatic. At the time, doctors told them the "truth" as best they knew it. The accepted medical fact until the mid-1980s was that if you had breast cancer, you had to undergo a radical mastectomy to remove your breast as well as the dissection of the lymph nodes under your arm, which often caused your arm to become permanently swollen and nonfunctional. The overall self-esteem of these women plunged and their feelings about themselves as women were often damaged beyond repair.

One patient's husband refused to allow his wife to undress in front of him even though it had been many years since she had had the mastectomy. This was so upsetting to her that she even contemplated undergoing expensive and drastic reconstructive surgery. In those days, doctors believed that if these women did not have radical surgery, they would lose their lives. The current "truth" is that lumpectomy—removing only the lump from the affected breast—is equally effective. And so the devastating truth that all those women were told is no longer the truth.

There is never just one truth. There are a great many truths. There's a truth for the doctor and a different truth for each and every patient. And so this idea of *"I want my doctor to tell me the truth"* is an oversimplification. Physicians are obliged to answer any questions a patient has as well as they can. I know physicians who lie awake nights worrying about whether their level of knowledge about a particular patient's health problem is adequate to constitute the absolute truth. All any doctor can offer is expertise, experience, and judgment.

If there are ten patients who did very well on a certain treatment, for example, this does not justify the delusion of thinking that all patients will always do equally well with that treatment. But if, as a doctor, I feel comfortable using that treatment because I have been successful helping patients, then that's my truth. On the other hand, if a patient is reluctant to take a certain medication because he knows someone who took the same thing and suffered terribly, then that's his truth. His reluctance should be respected. So both patients and doctors have their own truths.

When you feel you have not gotten enough information from your doctor, ask questions! Patients, friends, and families should be encouraged to ask questions when they feel the need to know more. It forces doctors not only to face the issues with patients, but also to come to grips with it themselves.

In the case of Mrs. W., who had been told that her premature baby had only a 20 percent chance of survival, when her baby did in fact survive, she was faced with some complicated decisions. In the days when large amounts of oxygen were used to help premature babies survive, they sometimes developed a serious eye disease known as retro-lental hyperplasia. This unfortunate baby developed the disease and the retinas were beginning to detach. Mrs. W. was then asked to decide whether she wanted her baby to have surgery. The surgeon did not give her enough information and she did not push him to tell her more. She was offered two options: to have corrective surgery or simply wait and see how her baby would do without surgery. He did not make it clear to her that a time factor was involved; the longer she took to arrive at a decision, the greater the possibility that the problem would become more severe or even inoperable. In a later interview, I asked what she remembered about the decisions she was asked to make. She answered in her broken English, becoming upset at the recollection:

> MRS. W.: *Well, first time they ask me to ah, she has an eye problem because she is premature, they using the oxygen . . . that retina detached, so they like to open the eye. They said it's up to you. Then I have the choice just to close my eye—the choice I wish to good luck. That was, ah, you know, still I feel that they hold my neck.*

Here she explains to me that, because of the detached retina, her doctors wanted to *"open,"* or perform surgery on her baby's eye. The surgeons then dropped the decision entirely in her lap. She only had the choice, she says, to close her eyes and leave it to luck. But all the while, she felt as if the doctors were forcing her into a decision: *"They hold my neck."*

> DR. KORSCH: *They put it all on you.*
>
> MRS. W: *Then I tell the answer—"Yes, go ahead." It's been taking two weeks.*
>
> DR. KORSCH: *To think?*
>
> MRS. W: *Yes. Then after they came out from the operating room, doctor say it's complete—almost completely detached, so they cannot do anything else. And as time is passed before me. Now I'm thinking that I was stupid, I spent two weeks.*

Here she tells me that it took her two weeks to finally make a decision. And it was not until after the surgery that the doctor told her that she had waited too long, that the retinas were beyond repair. Now she feels that everything is her fault, *"I was stupid."*

> DR. KORSCH: *You feel stupid?*
>
> MRS. W.: *Yes. Thinking. But nobody asked me, or told me—"We need it rush," or "Why are you holding it too long."... Nobody didn't say if we do it in little time, you know, only then....*
>
> DR. KORSCH: *Might be better.*
>
> MRS. W.: *Might be better. Nobody didn't say. Everybody quiet.*

She tells me that no one told her that there was a rush, no one asked her why she was waiting so long. No one told her that there was only a limited time in which to make a decision.

I talked to her about why she didn't ask her doctors more questions:

> MRS. W.: *But, uh, I didn't give to them any questions. Not any questions.... Because most of people, they don't want to answer, exactly, you know.*

DR. KORSCH: *Do you think if you ask, people don't like it? Do you feel they don't trust?*

MRS. W.: *No. I think they like to talk but they don't want to have responsibility of what they're talking.*

DR. KORSCH: *Mmm. So you figure you better not ask.*

MRS. W.: *Yes.*

This mother's plight poignantly demonstrates that we can't always rely on our doctors to take the initiative to communicate. Consequently, it is often up to us to challenge our doctors to give us enough information so we can make informed decisions. In most settings, doctor and patient benefit.

Why Patients Don't Tell the Truth

Let's turn the tables. Doctors aren't the only ones who withhold information. Have you ever not told your doctor the truth? When patients are not completely honest, they risk their own health. If you choose not to tell your doctor about certain things, you are taking risks that your health care will suffer. If there are things that you hesitate to discuss with your doctor, ask yourself why. It may be because you think that if you tell the doctor, he or she might judge you harshly. As patients, it shouldn't be our priority to impress our doctors with how wonderful we are. We want them to take care of us when we're down, when we're in trouble, and perhaps even when we've done things we're ashamed of.

But we know that physicians have likes and dislikes and personal opinions, and we naturally make an effort to come across positively. When I go to doctors, I can't help trying to impress them with how strong and positive I am and I try to engage them so that they will like me. That's human and almost universal. Whenever we meet new people, whether in a professional setting or at a social gathering, most of us naturally try to look good. And when we meet a physician who is going to examine and treat us, our need to impress is intensified.

We entrust physicians to make important decisions for us and sometimes we have to place our lives in their hands. To start with, we are at a disadvantage in the relationship. We have to expose ourselves physically and emotionally in a way that challenges our self-esteem. We are especially eager then to make them like us, even though they are seeing us at our worst. The doctor doesn't need to impress us because he or she is the one with the knowledge, the clothes, and the power. That's what makes us feel that we must make our doctors like us, even though it's not part of the official contract. Most patients do feel, probably inappropriately, that getting the best treatment will partly depend on whether the doctor likes them.

If you feel obliged to come across as the I-*can-take-it, I'll-do-anything-you-say* patient, you may find yourself unable to discuss your problems honestly. If you can't be honest, there is something wrong with the relationship. You should never feel that you have to seduce your physician into giving you good care by pretending that you don't hurt. If you have been holding back, perhaps hesitating to admit, for instance, that you did not follow the instructions you were given during your last visit, then test the relationship. Tell your doctor and observe the response while listening carefully. Your doctor should react sensitively and you should feel better after listening to his or her reply. This is a good way of judging the resiliency of the relationship and of exploring what kinds of stresses it can tolerate.

If there are things you want to know, then ask! If there are certain things you do not want to know, don't think that you have to live up to the *I'm-tough, give-it-to-me-straight* image simply because you think the doctor will admire you for it. It's your choice. You have a right to expect that your doctor will not make judgments about you or consider you a coward. This is another excellent way to test your relationship. If you hesitate to tell your doctor to protect you from painful information for fear he will respect you less, then reevaluate whether you are overreacting or whether your doctor actually is that judgmental. You should be completely comfortable saying,

> *"I really don't want to hear all the details—I can only handle so much information at a time. Please tell me what I need to know right now so that I can make my decisions and then I'll come back to you with questions."*

This is a good way of finding out whether your doctor is right for you. If you are uncomfortable and believe the doctor is, in fact, judging you, it doesn't mean that he is a bad doctor. It may just mean that you are misinterpreting. There is no reason why you can't sit down with the doctor and say,

> *"You know, I came to you because you're highly recommended and I have a lot of confidence in you. I know you're technically competent and I like the way you treat me, but I find myself hesitant to tell you some of my fears because I'm afraid of what you will think. Could we work on that together?"*

If you are still not satisfied, then it may mean that you need to find another doctor with whom you can negotiate freely.

Have you ever caught yourself telling your doctor something that you realized was not quite the truth? It has been documented over and over that some people even go to psychiatrists to get help, pay hundreds of dollars per session, and then tell lies. A physician considering divorce went to a psychiatrist for a few sessions. He later told me,

> *"I needed to make sure, within myself, that I wasn't making a terrible mistake by leaving my wife. After a few sessions, I realized how much I had been covering up. In talking about some of the things that had happened, I had provided excuses, usually in a way to make myself look better. And so I went back and said, 'What I told you really wasn't the way it was at the time . . . she didn't actually say it the way I told you . . . it was I who was so furious . . . that may be the reason she acted the way she did.'"*

There is no doubt that it's very tempting to present yourself in a more positive light even when it is definitely not in your own interests. The psychiatrist he visited was not there to judge him, she was there to help him solve the dilemma. But his response to the situation shows how much he needed to deceive himself to preserve his image.

What is it about going to the doctor that keeps us from being completely truthful? We don't do it deliberately; often it is just because we cannot bring ourselves to talk about what is bothering us. It's human nature. We even fool ourselves in our own memories. What the physician presented to the psychiatrist was his current version of reality. It actually took him a few sessions to realize he had been deceiving himself as well as the doctor.

We all have been guilty of not telling the truth or at least not telling all of the truth at one time or another. We may emphasize things that are not that important and suppress others that are significant. Very few relationships are completely honest. At one point or another, we have all been dishonest with others and perhaps even ourselves in relationships and different life situations.

We must be as open in communication with our physicians as possible if we want help based on the reality of our situation. Let's take a simple example. Suppose you want to stop smoking. You go to the doctor and explain that you really are highly motivated to quit. He tells you to start chewing gum when you feel like having a cigarette, to avoid high-risk situations where you are more likely to get the urge, and suggests that at work, if your stress level is mounting, it might be better to walk around the block than to reach for a cigarette. He also prescribes a nicotine patch to help you in your struggle. He tells you how well these have worked for some of his patients and how successful many of them have been in kicking the habit. Even while he is explaining what you are expected to do, you begin to have grave doubts. You mislead him because you don't want to admit that you don't trust yourself to do it.

As you anticipated, it proves difficult for you to carry out the doctor's instructions. You find that it's easy to apply the patch, but impossible to cut out the cigarettes. Now, you become progressively more embarrassed and may even avoid going back to the doctor because you are ashamed. You would have been better off telling your doctor at the outset why some of his instructions could not possibly work. You may hate chewing gum, the social situations where people smoke may be unavoidable, and it may not be practical for you to leave your office every time you have the urge to smoke. You're also afraid of gaining the extra weight that some people pick up when they stop smoking. If you had spoken up, you and the physician might have been able to work out a more realistic plan.

Have you ever wanted to tell your doctor something, but were afraid of offending him by questioning his advice? I had a patient who was a paramedic and had an accident that injured his leg. While he was hospitalized for treatment, he noticed that when the nurses were changing his dressing, there were breaks in the sterile technique that might contaminate his wound. He told me that he held back his questions and critical comments from the doctors and also the nurses for fear that he would offend them. He mentioned that after he had, in fact, criticized something that a nurse had done, it would take the nurse longer to come to his bedside when he called. He wondered whether even the fact that his dinner tray was delivered late and the food was no longer hot might have been a consequence of his having spoken up. He told me that he was disgusted that he had to be so diplomatic to get optimal treatment, but he did learn to be careful with his criticism in the future.

What Can Patients Do?

Patients are dependent on doctors for good treatment. Although you shouldn't have to use diplomacy to get proper care, it is difficult—in fact nearly impossible—to lay down rules governing what patients can do. It really is a judgment call. When you realize that there is a significant issue you would like to discuss, yet fear how your doctor would react, you certainly need to raise it. Tell yourself,

> *I really do need to inform him [or her] because it might affect my treatment.*

You are basically taking the responsibility for the communication breakdown. Assume ownership of the problem instead of blaming the doctor for your fears. Chances are the doctor will not be offended. This is another excellent test of the relationship, so watch and see how your doctor reacts.

Doctors are not the only important members of the health-care team from whom patients withhold information. Nowadays, the doctor is but a small part of the whole process. There are receptionists, office managers, nurses, physicians' assistants, and medical technicians who become every bit as important in the communication process as the doctors themselves. They can be extremely helpful or, when things go badly, they can become barriers that hinder us in achieving the communication we want with our doctors.

Years ago, when I'd call a doctor's office in reference to a patient and the person answering the phone asked what my call was about, I'd get on my high horse and simply cut her out of the communication process. As a doctor, I wanted to speak with the doctor and I didn't want to spend time getting into lengthy explanations. Now, I've learned to give the maximum information to all members of the health-care team. If the assistant asks me for further information, whether it's about my own health or a conference about a patient, I explain as much as possible. Why? Because by sharing the information, I'm empowering the assistant and she becomes my partner. But if I say, *"No, this is something I can only talk to the doctor about,"* then I have made an enemy who feels put down and is less motivated to help.

In your own communication with the health-care team, being open can only improve the services you receive. Be honest with yourself about why you hesitate to talk about certain things. Make sure that in your next encounter, even though you may still be ashamed or embarrassed, you will nevertheless be able to raise the issue:

> *"There are some things I should have told you last time but I found myself embarrassed. And I don't really know why. I have trouble telling you about it but it may be important for you to know so that you can understand me better."*

Who Owns the Information About Your Health?

It is the law that patients have the right to have access to medical information about themselves. That does not, however, mean that we can always have the right to directly and completely review our own medical records. It is actually up to each particular physician's discretion exactly how much medical information a patient gets and how it will be interpreted. While only you can authorize the transfer or release of your medical records, it is at the physician's discretion how much information will actually be sent. Your physician may decide to withhold some aspects of the information about you if he or she believes that it is not in your best interests or that it could be detrimental to the doctor–patient relationship.

In a functional doctor–patient relationship, you should feel that your doctor is giving you adequate information about your health and your care. If not, you should ask your doctor to inform you more completely. When a patient starts worrying about how to get access to information, that may be a sign of communication breakdown. Before requesting legal access to your records, it is a good idea to discuss with your physician why you need them and whether you are dissatisfied about the way he or she has been informing you.

Although the legalities of accessing our records seem forbidding, in most instances if you simply ask your doctor, chances are he or she will have no objection. Try it! Doctors often just assume that we are uninterested. In fact, many patients don't look even when they have the opportunity. You have probably never set eyes on those information-packed, sacred pages, and, although you may have trouble understanding what's there, it may afford you an occasion to ask questions.

A few years ago, a colleague told me about a patient, Jim, a college professor, who was involved in a lawsuit because of an automobile accident in which he sustained several fractures. At his lawyer's request, Jim asked his orthopedist for the X rays, but the doctor refused to hand them over. Weeks went by while the doctor and lawyer attempted to communicate by phone, and Jim grew more and more frustrated. When Jim finally returned to his doctor's office and demanded the X rays, the orthopedist insisted that only he could give the information to the lawyer and that only he would discuss the findings with him. Jim said that since there was so much "telephone tag" going on between the three, it would be easiest if he could just take the X rays to the lawyer himself. The doctor became increasingly annoyed because he resented having Jim tell him what to do. By instructing the doctor to give him the X rays, Jim was actually threatening his doctor's power. Who was right? Should the doctor have handed them over? Did Jim have the right to demand that they be handed over?

Too Much Information?

There may be times when having all the available information about ourselves may not be in our own best interests and could actually be harmful. While on the one hand, we're making progress in terms of having physicians be much more open to giving information and patients having more access to it in general, on the other hand, we're creating new problems. The explosion of technical knowledge has severe implications for our daily lives as well as our health care.

Almost every day new discoveries in genetics tell us whether we are more likely to die from high blood pressure, stroke, or cancer. A recent study involving a genetic test to identify patients who are susceptible to breast cancer showed that not all patients wanted the test.[7] So information is being uncovered that, although you are entitled to it, has implications that you may not wish to learn. A record of the fact that you are predisposed to certain diseases may put you at risk for not getting health-care insurance as easily. In some cases you can take appropriate measures; in others you cannot. Things get more and more complex as technology continues to expand.

The following controversial case raised such important questions about the ownership of information that it had to be evaluated by the hospital ethics committee. It was a real puzzle to everyone. What do *you* think would have been the right thing to do?

The family of a child needing a bone-marrow transplant was tested to find out who would be the best donor. In the course of the testing, it became apparent that the mother's husband was not the patient's biological father. This unexpected discovery posed some difficult questions for the doctors. It was known that the child's disease could only be passed along if both parents had traits for it. The "father" believed that he had the trait for the disease, which we then knew was not the case. This information was significant and he deserved to know it in case he planned to have other children.

How much information were the doctors obliged to give to the patient's family? And what was the "father" entitled to be told? There were endless discussions about whether the information should be given to the family and, if so, to whom. Should the doctors tell the mother and let her choose whether to discuss it with her husband? Should they not relay the information at all because that was not what the testing was officially done for? Should the doctors tell the mother and insist that she tell her husband and cause possibly serious family disruption? Should they tell the "father" directly? To whom did the information belong? One member of the group felt that the whole problem lay in not having gotten informed consent from the family prior to the testing. He thought they should have been told:

> *"From this test, we may discover things about your family's genetics that have nothing to do with what we are looking for. Would you like to be completely informed about all of the results?"*

Another member of the committee, a hematologist, was up in arms at that suggestion. He said:

> *"If we have to tell that to every patient who is being cross-matched, even just for a blood transfusion, and it turns out that they are not the father of their children, we're never going to be able to get blood anymore! Would that be in the best interests of our patients?"*

In retrospect, a sensitive and complete family history before the procedure might have revealed that the "father" was not the biological father.

How would you have solved this dilemma? At what point is it appropriate to give a patient information that might be disturbing? Is it best to tell a patient what you, as a doctor, may learn no matter what? And if you learn something about your patients that has nothing to do with what you were originally looking for, are you committed to tell them?

In the end, this patient's mother agreed that both parents should be informed and, fortunately, the marriage did not seem to suffer. The father, it turned out, already knew that the patient was not his own child and was content to have the information about his blood type and inheritance. In this case and in certain others, it is really the patient's responsibility to give relevant information to the doctor. This makes for a better relationship, better health care and, in fact, has been determined to be the patient's duty. In a malpractice case, for instance, if you have withheld important information from your doctor, it can count against you.

Who Has the Power?

From the moment we walk into an examination room and begin to take off our clothes, it is almost as if we are abdicating our power and relegating it to another person. No matter how smart, how educated, or how wise we are, when we sit on that table, nude under the skimpy paper coverup, waiting expectantly for the all-knowing doctor, it becomes difficult to feel very powerful. Everyone in the office, from nurses to assistants, tells us what to do and what not to do, usually without exploring our preferences or even explaining why.

Despite of our eagerness to make autonomous decisions, we still must delegate a lot of power to the doctor. As patients, we continually find ourselves feeling helpless and humiliated. The traditional doctor–patient relationship involves an imbalance and most of the power resides with the physician. If the orthopedist who refused to relinquish the X rays to the patient had actually released them, the patient would have been in a stronger position. But, the doctor did not hand over the records and the patient's struggle to have a little power failed.

Ideally, information should reside with the responsible patient. This person should have the power to own the information, take control of it, and decide who's going to hear what. There has been quite a lot of discussion lately that we, as patients, should be the captain of the health-care team because, after all, it's our body and we have the right to make the decisions. But to what extent this idea can be acted on in real life is an interesting question. Although you may be the legal owner of all the information about yourself, it is sometimes not quite that easy. The doctor makes the decision about the flow of information, and when a doctor's judgment and decisions are based on the patient's best interests, there is no problem. But there is also the risk of doctors withholding information as a power ploy. In fact, information sharing has been one of the features of the doctor–patient interaction that has played a central role in the transition from a patriarchal, authoritarian relationship toward a more equal partnership in which the patient is an increasingly active participant.

What happens when the physician becomes the patient? Does the physician as patient also have to abdicate power? Not long ago, a physician I know had a biopsy of a questionable spot on his skin. The dermatologist who did the biopsy said,

"I'll call you if there is something to worry about."

The patient heard nothing for two weeks and, being a doctor, hesitated to call his doctor because she had said that she would contact him if something were up. The idea of "No news is good news" is infinite and ambiguous. Patients want to hear the doctor say,

"The results were negative—you're fine."

It was three weeks after the biopsy when the patient stepped into a crowded hospital elevator and spotted his dermatologist among the crowd. That's when he heard the bad news: *"Oh, I've been meaning to call you,"* she broadcasted, *"I was right, that lesion was malignant."* She had the information about the patient for at least two weeks and yet had withheld it. The patient later commented: *"And I had been hesitant to call her because I had not wanted to seem too pushy. I'll never recommend her again!"*

So even though the patient was actually a doctor, the relationship had shifted. The unique doctor–patient relationship had caused a reluctance on the patient's part to make a justifiable inquiry for fear that the treating doctor would be offended. The very fact that the dermatologist had performed the surgery and had access to the biopsy information created a power imbalance. This prevented the patient from insisting on a timely report. Once the physician was defined as a patient, he felt powerless and hesitant to demand the information he was entitled to.

The more we know about our health, the more autonomous and capable we become in decision making. It is undoubtedly true that if you feel you have been deceived by a doctor, you will lose trust. The physician-patient in the last example certainly did not return to the dermatologist because, as he put it,

> *"I felt angry that she had not told me sooner, humiliated that she had chosen to give me the news in front of an elevator full of people, and uneasy that she had known the lab results for quite some time without telling me. I lost my trust in her."*

If you have all the information you need and know your contingencies, you have more control over your own life. To illustrate this for my trainees, I use an analogy from everyday family life. If a little boy says, *"Mom can we go to the movies tonight?"* and she says, *"We'll see,"* then she's keeping all the power and he has no control. He has to wait, suspended with no options, to see what will happen. But if instead she says, *"If Daddy gets home from work early and if you help get dinner on the table and help with the dishes and we get through in time, then I think we might be able to go,"* then the child has knowledge of the contingencies and of several ways he can control the situation.

The same principle applies in medicine. If a patient is recovering from a minor stroke and has high blood pressure and asks,

"What is the likelihood I'll have another stroke?"

If the doctor's answer is something like,

"If you reduce the salt in your diet, control your blood pressure with the medication I'm prescribing, and are reasonable about the amount of extra activity you do, then chances are that you may never have another one,"

then the patient is informed and empowered. He can try to keep himself healthy. This is psychologically better for him and may even improve his prognosis. Doctors who take the opposite approach are like the parent who gave the child no control: *"Well, we'll see."* That leaves the patient hanging without options.

We yearn for someone whom we can trust. On the one hand, we complain that doctors are too patronizing and that they should not be able to decide how much information we should have, but, on the other hand, we don't want to rob them of their power to help us. That's what's so tricky. I have traces of a patronizing, patriarchal physician in me and I also personally feel the need for that kind of physician when I visit a doctor. The current trend is for the maximum amount of information sharing, which empowers the patient and makes the patient a partner. But when it comes to my own health, I'm not so sure I want to be a partner with my doctor. I do want to be a well-educated, informed patient and I do not want to be lied to. Yet, I want someone who is going to help me, protect me, and take care of me.

The next time you visit your doctor, increased knowledge of your options may aid you in feeling more powerful. This applies not only to the big decisions about your medical care, but also to your everyday experiences in the office. For instance, when the nurse shows you into the exam room and requests that you undress, you can politely challenge her by requesting that she give you her best estimate on how long it will be until the doctor is ready to see you. You may learn, for instance, that the doctor had an emergency earlier in the day that put him behind schedule. This means you will have to wait. If you find out that he is ten minutes behind schedule, you then have enough information to exert some control over your situation. You may choose to wait eight minutes before getting undressed. If your doctor is running behind by a half hour and you have limited time, you may decide to reschedule your appointment. If you are making a first visit to a doctor's office, ask to be introduced to the physician while you are still fully dressed, before the examination begins, so as to retain as much dignity and power as possible. I encourage women who are visiting a gynecologist to request that the nurse inform them when the doctor is ready to see them so that they don't have to wait for what seems like hours in that most humiliating of all positions.

Who empowers whom and under what circumstances? Among professionals nowadays, it's fashionable to talk about "empowering" the patient. This is really a very patronizing concept because the patient already has the power. Instead of "empowering" the patient, the only thing a physician can really do is restore the patient's power. It is, after all, the patient who seeks out the doctor. The patient can always walk out or refuse. So the underlying power structure is that the patient is in charge. Nevertheless, in certain patient–physician relationships, the power is, in large measure, taken away from the patient. But we don't always have to accept that.

As a doctor, I ask myself how I can assess what an individual patient can and wants to handle. I can ask the patient how much she wants to know. Although that is a very important step, the trouble is that it can be misleading because patients want to please their doctors. They perceive that their doctors like patients who are strong and brave. So my patient may ask questions to impress me without realizing or being prepared for the kind of information I will give. If I go by the law—that I must obtain a completely informed consent—I may literally scare my patient to death. On the other hand, I am obliged to share the information.

As patients, we do have the full right to have information and to criticize doctors who withhold it rendering us less able to make decisions about our lives. But nothing in life is that simple. Giving the maximum amount of information is not always best. There is always a medical truth, a human truth, and medical ethics to consider. The question is, should there be an absolute rule that doctors must not lie? There will always be the one instance in which deceiving may be right. When you're dealing with human beings and tricky issues, nothing is absolute. As a physician, I'm no longer as ready to accept the idea that the information we give honestly to our patients is always the truth. Patients need to be aware that medical science is not always perfect. They need to know that their physicians will attempt to inform them as well as they can, but that an honest physician cannot pretend to know the absolute and final truth.

DOES YOUR DOCTOR
SEEM UNFEELING?

Have you ever visited a doctor, talked about something that was really bothering you, and ended up feeling dissatisfied because your physician did not seem to react to your concerns? Perhaps your doctor was listening, standing up, with no facial expression, and made only matter-of-fact recommendations. Or concentrated on writing notes on a clipboard, never making eye contact with you. Maybe the doctor shrugged off your concerns by saying, *"Relax, don't worry about it,"* treating them as if *you* were overreacting.

We would all like our doctors to let us know that they understand. When they don't, we lose confidence in our treatment:

> *"If my doctor doesn't even care about how bad I feel, how is he going to be able to help me?"*

You go to the doctor because you feel sick and need help. The doctor is there as a professional and is feeling perfectly well. You, naturally, are anxious and perhaps are nervously dreading your appointment. The physician, neither anxious nor nervous, is there to perform a task. You are all alone. The doctor is aided by a health-care team of assistants, nurses, and perhaps even other doctors. You may feel helpless, even disempowered. The doctor has all the power. You are unprepared for the encounter. The doctor has spent a good part of his or her life preparing. You and your doctor each have a completely different mind-set. You want help and reassurance. The doctor needs to make a diagnosis and treat your illness; responding to your feelings is not his highest priority.

When I have asked patients whether they would rather have a doctor who is kind or one who is a good technician, it rarely occurs to them to say that they would like to have one with both qualities. In their minds, a highly competent physician is also less likely to be empathetic. Some say all they want is a doctor who will do the best job. Others become resentful if the doctor seems matter-of-fact and task oriented.

I encourage physicians-in-training to be more empathetic and more open, but they frequently become defensive—*"I haven't got the time. . . . I can't sit down and cry with every patient!"*

When I recently presented my ideas on the doctor–patient relationship to a symposium of distinguished physicians, they articulately resisted what I had to say and informed me, *"We are here to take care of sick patients; we don't have time for that sentimental stuff."* One physician in my hostile audience stood up and told an anecdote about a resident who was so preoccupied with her patients' feelings that she sat down and held the hand of a patient in cardiac arrest instead of treating the acute problems. For my audience on that day, a doctor could be either empathic or competent, but not both. Even when I approach my own medical students and interns to discuss more sensitive ways of handling certain situations, I often find them ambivalent. They have grown up in a culture in which the doctor–patient relationship and effective communication are not part of the science of medicine.

Of course, there are times when a patient chooses a doctor for a specific skill alone and is not concerned, at first, with whether the doctor expresses empathy and can communicate well. Patients often select surgeons and other highly specialized physicians because they have heard of their technical expertise. I chose my internist because he was competent and conscientious. I trusted him completely and I went to him for years, but he was not really concerned with anything except the hard medical facts. At the time when my husband Robert was dying of cancer, my family began to worry about me and urged me to go in for a checkup of my own. The doctor examined me right after he had seen my husband. He knew that Robert was desperately ill, in the final stages of cancer, and that I was caring for him at home. While listening to my heart, he began to look puzzled, then queried, *"You have some premature heartbeats there that you didn't have before. . . . Have you been under any stress lately?"*

He had asked me a question that, under other circumstances, might have been appropriate. But given my situation, it struck me as highly insensitive. Had I been under any stress lately? My dying husband was his patient. I replied indignantly, *"Well, you've just seen Robert, of course I've been under stress!"*

On another occasion, the same physician spent an unusual amount of time carefully examining my abdomen. With no explanation, he sent me down to have a "flat-plate" taken. The radiologist took what seemed like an unusually long time in setting up for this procedure, making precise measurements of the distance between the X ray camera and my abdomen. I knew this was not routine and that he must be looking for something specific. My anxiety mounted. Lying on the table, I imagined all sorts of terrible things about what could possibly be wrong. Had he felt a tumor? If I had cancer, who would take care of my husband when I had to go to the hospital? When I later saw the doctor in his consultation room, I asked him what was going on. He responded on a positive note, *"Oh, you're fine,"* he said, *"but you know, I've had some very good luck recently diagnosing abdominal aneurysms in several of my patients . . . you had rather strong pulsations so I thought I'd take an X ray to see if you had one."* I couldn't help thinking about the other poor patients who had certainly not been lucky. Did he think that it would actually make me feel better to know how "lucky" he had been in making the correct diagnosis and that he had suspected that I also might have an aneurysm?

Doctors do have insensitive ways of responding to patients' anxieties. Sometimes they make humorous statements intended to be funny but which fall flat and even come across as callous. By making light of emotions and trying to amuse patients, they are often able to bypass their own feelings. Overweight patients are jokingly referred to as "skinny," older female patients addressed as "young lady." While checking an elderly patient's poor eyesight, the surgeon quipped, *"You're lucky you're not a pilot."*

One patient who was facing serious surgery and was extremely frightened told me that her physician, instead of giving her a reassuring explanation of the procedure, quipped, *"Oh, in spite of all this, you'll still bury me!"*

A young medical student I know was having a plantar wart removed from the bottom of her foot under a local anesthetic. While the surgeon was performing the minor operation, he sang the old song, *"You'll never smile again . . . ,"* but substituted the word "dance" for smile. The patient was not amused.

While I have heard countless patient complaints about doctors who "don't care," those physicians who try to be extra sympathetic do not always get rave reviews either. I referred an acquaintance to a pediatrician who was highly skilled and competent but who was also sensitive and interested in patients as people. About a year later, she called me back and asked me to recommend another doctor. When I asked her why, she replied, *"Oh, I don't know, all he ever does is pat me on the back, tell me I'm doing a good job . . . he's very kind but I just don't feel confident."*

I later found out that he had worried that she was anxious and unsure of herself as a mother and, as a result, he had devoted a lot of time to addressing her thoughts and feelings about that during their medical encounters. Although he had never made an error with any of the technical tasks in caring for her child, his strategy of focusing on her feelings undermined her confidence in him as a physician.

Ideally, we all would like our physicians to be completely dedicated. In the best of all worlds, our doctors would cater to all our needs and we would no longer have any complaints. Although that sort of an arrangement does seem alluring, it doesn't work. When physicians consistently go beyond what should realistically be expected of them, they become less responsive to their patients. *"If you see fifty patients in a day,"* one physician commented, *"all of whom have real problems, and the fifty-first breaks down and cries, you are no longer able to be truly empathic."*

The Last Angry Man, a book published in 1941, tells the story of a self-sacrificing physician who made himself available to his patients night and day, seven days a week, and stopped at nothing to help them. Not only did he care for their medical problems, he also responded to many other requests. He sacrificed every waking moment of his life and all his energy to taking care of his patients. This caused him to feel that no matter how grateful his patients were, it could never be enough to reward and repay him for his services. For the patients, it became a complex relationship. They hesitated to make their complaints known—and add to his burdens. It was uncomfortable for them to owe their doctor that much gratitude.

This problem applies, in varying extents, to doctor–patient relationships today. Physicians put in extra long days, are on call twenty-four hours, and naturally feel entitled to gratitude—this, in turn, makes their patients feel obligated. There are still physicians who go beyond the call of duty by literally doing everything for their patients—filling out paperwork, giving personal advice, procuring household help, acquiring medications wholesale, helping them find a place to live, and so on. Sometimes this kind of devotion is at the physician's own expense, sometimes it's at the expense of their family, and in other instances, they unconsciously extract the price from their patients. The patients of these totally giving physicians may even hesitate in being honest. They feel they owe a tremendous emotional debt. They do not want to disappoint their doctors in any way by their own weakness.

Can Someone Who Has Never Been Sick Be a Good Doctor?

When patients are discouraged in the way they are treated by their physicians and feel their doctors are not empathic, they sometimes attribute it to the fact that the doctor has not had the same malady and has no idea what it is *really* like. It is not uncommon to hope that the doctor knows exactly how we feel, but if you make the assumption that your doctor will be more empathetic because he or she had a similar experience, you may find yourself disappointed. In fact, doctors who have had the same ailments as their patients are often perceived as being *less* helpful! Physicians who have gone through an illness or injury and use themselves as an illustration may actually irritate patients and end up coming across as uncaring.

The doctor may have found a solution to his own problem, but patients may end up resentful because it does not work for them. If you are trying to lose weight and your doctor says, *"Oh I'd picked up a little weight too, so I started working out and eating less. My cholesterol was down in three months and now I'm having no trouble keeping my weight down,"* you may not be as thrilled by his success story as he is. When you have tried the same thing and failed, facing your doctor, who has been successful, can be really exasperating.

When a patient, Mary Ann, developed a painful bursitis of the elbow, she consulted her doctor and learned that he had experienced a similar problem. In light of this, she was surprised when he was not at all empathetic toward her. *"I had the same thing,"* he lightheartedly reassured her, *"and after a few weeks I was just fine."* That seemed encouraging at first. During her following visits, when she was not improving as fast, Mary Ann felt there must definitely be something wrong. The doctor had been able to conquer his own problem rapidly and she felt that this was the reason he had no sympathy for her persistent symptoms.

One time, when Mary Ann began asking questions about how soon she would regain normal function, he ignored her question and quipped, *"Don't worry about your elbow, just worry about your new job!"* Mary Ann needed to talk about her level of activity and when she could get back to her normal routine. She had taken time off from her job to go to the appointment, driven an hour during the morning rush hour to get there, and needed more information. His comment literally stopped her in her tracks. She was silent for the remainder of the visit, did not ask any more questions, and in fact did not return for her follow-up appointment.

How distressed should our doctors be about our illnesses? Can they understand without becoming equally distressed themselves? Many doctors believe that they have only two alternatives: either go to pieces and suffer too much with the patient, which is damaging to both physician and patient, or simply suppress feelings all together, which limits how helpful they can be.

Most of us do want our doctors to care, but if they become overinvolved they may not be as supportive, strong, and able to give us the care we need. In studies conducted to explore patients' responses to the manner in which they had been given bad news, it was found that doctors used two different approaches.[1] One involved the doctor being matter-of-fact, abrupt, and almost cruel in giving the information. The opposite approach had the physician being so sympathetic that he almost broke down and cried with the patient. Neither approach satisfied patients. The doctors who had been abrupt had offended and further upset their patients. Those who had become emotional were not perceived by patients as a source of sufficient strength. The patients may have appreciated the sympathy, but did not feel as if they were receiving enough help or support.

As the patient, it is up to you to establish the tenor of the relationship. The doctor is prepared and confident for the encounter, and you should do your level best to also be as prepared and confident as possible. Formulate an agenda. If the doctor is not sensitive or skilled enough to elicit what you want to talk about and respond to your feelings, there is no one else who can make it a part of the agenda except you. Speak up:

"There are a couple of things that are really worrying me . . . ."

If you find that the doctor is not sufficiently responsive when you complain of pain or other symptoms, the next move is yours. If your doctor glosses over the subject and says something like, *"What I'd really like to do today is adjust the dosage of your blood pressure medication,"* then hold your ground.

Watch out for becoming too emotional or aggressive because it will cause the doctor to get defensive. But insist:

"I realize that's very important, but before we finish our visit today, there are a couple of really urgent questions I haven't had the chance to bring up. The things that are really bothering me the most are _____ ."

If, despite your efforts, you have gained no ground, there are still a few alternatives. First, you can politely say, *"I need the chance to talk to someone about what is bothering me. If you don't have the time today, should I make another appointment?"*

Another option is to talk to the office nurse or an assistant:

"The doctor was very busy today and I did not get the chance to talk about some of my concerns. I would really like to hear what she thinks. Should I call her later?"

In most instances, the nurse will offer to listen to your questions, may be able to give you helpful information, and can either have the doctor call you later or telephone you herself after conferring with the doctor about your concerns.

A young woman who has recently been found to have cancer goes to a doctor who treats her illness, but never gives her the opportunity to speak up. She feels that she is not being treated like an individual and has complained that she has been given little, if any, chance to discuss things that are bothering her. After a number of failed attempts to break through this communication barrier, she finally gathers her courage:

> *"You keep talking about my cancer as if it's just one more of your biopsy reports from the lab. You are giving me nothing but these terrible options for treatment and you don't seem to be aware that I'm young and had no idea until a few weeks ago that there was anything wrong with me at all.*
>
> *"What should I do? All this information is frightening—I can't even listen anymore.*
>
> *"I really need some help in accepting this . . . . I need to come in with my husband so we can discuss this together."*

In less than twenty-five seconds, this patient politely but firmly conveyed her concerns about her situation and the way she was being treated.

Are You in Pain or Just Uncomfortable?

Have you ever tried to tell your doctor how much something hurts and felt ignored and of little importance to the doctor? Pain is subjective. There is no way a physician can "feel" a patient's pain. In an attempt to measure your pain, your doctor may ask you to rate it on a scale of 1 to 10, but that can be cold comfort when you are suffering. Besides, doctors will not always accept your estimate of how much it hurts and tend to make their own decisions. In fact, doctors do not like it when patients complain. Again and again, I hear physicians say, *"He's complaining a lot, but it doesn't really hurt that much."* They appreciate patients who are brave and cheerfully say, *"I can take it, I'm doing great, thank you."*

When a patient feels pain, the doctor does not. And so, when a doctor tells a patient, *"It won't really hurt, but you may just be a little uncomfortable,"* many patients, because they are too embarrassed, hesitate to complain even though they are hurting. The doctor is trying to be objective but he or she has no way of really knowing the intensity of your pain.

As a visiting professor at a large teaching hospital, I noticed that some of the patients who were to undergo transplants were on dialysis longer than necessary. As time went by, these patients still had not undergone the operation. When I questioned the nursing staff, I learned that in some cases they had purposefully been delaying transplants for these patients. It was not, I was told, because the patients were not ready. It was because the transplant surgeon did not believe that pain medication was good for his patients. He thought it was inappropriate for them to complain after surgery because he really didn't think it hurt that much. And so he routinely avoided pain medications and his patients suffered without relief. The patients' reactions to their postoperative pain were so dramatic that the nonsurgical members of the team, who cared for them before and after surgery, became more and more reluctant to expose new patients to the same fate. And so certain transplants were actually delayed, keeping patients on dialysis.

There is a tremendous communication gap as to how patients perceive pain, how they expresses it, and the doctor's perception of the pain. Ironically, the more dramatic a patient becomes in describing pain,

"Oh, it's like a hammer banging on my forehead!"
"It feels like a knife turning in my chest!"

the more the doctor discounts it. And the more different the physician and patient are from one another, the fewer experiences they have in common, the less likely the physician will be to empathize with the pain. Menstrual cramps, for instance, have traditionally been thought of by male physicians (and by some female physicians who have not experienced painful cramps) as being purely psychological:

"It's all in your head."

Even labor pains have been debunked. Through the ages, this pain was regarded simply as an aspect of a woman's existence and she was expected not to complain too much and not to ask for medication. Even today, women are frequently looked down on, not empathized with, and treated as failures when they complain of pain or need medication during natural childbirth. In a sense, pain represents failure to physicians.

> *"Doctor, you are hurting me."*
> *"Doctor, you have not relieved my pain."*

These are words they don't like to hear. When a patient complains of pain, health professionals not uncommonly will observe, *"Oh, he's just carrying on . . . he's always so anxious."*

The dental office is a perfect example:

> *"This is just going to hurt a little bit and it will only take a couple of minutes so you're not going to need any Novocaine."*

How does the dentist know you won't need it? If you feel pain and if the doctor tells you that it doesn't really hurt that much, do not hesitate to speak up. Insist politely but firmly:

> *"Please listen to what I have to say. This is very important to me."*

Then, continue your approach with,

> *"There is no one except me who knows how much I hurt. Whether you think I should hurt this much or not is another question. It doesn't really help me at this moment if you think I should have had less pain or should be suffering less."*

If you're having an excruciating dental procedure, do not hesitate to say,

> *"I have a low pain threshold, and even though you think it may not hurt enough to require Novocaine, I do need it. I know myself and I can tolerate <u>very little pain</u>."*

It is your right to protest if the pain isn't relieved and you need *not* feel guilty about complaining. If your doctor hesitates to give you as much medication as you would like, then ask about alternative ways of alleviating the pain. If you are in the hospital after surgery, inquire whether they have a pain specialist. Don't wait too long to speak up—otherwise you'll set yourself up for an emotional encounter. And don't be overly emotional when describing pain. You're more likely to get attention if you don't attack the doctor because of the pain, but make an effort to calmly explain what you are feeling and what you would like done about it. If you go in with the attitude *"You're hurting me!,"* the doctor will become defensive and be more inclined to clam up. Approach the doctor with the attitude that you know he or she does want to help and that you would like the doctor to work with you:

> *"You've explained to me why you don't want to give too many drugs, but I would like to talk to you about what we can do when the pain is so bad. I'll do my best. If there is anything different I should be doing, I would like to know. But there are times when I do need relief."*

How to Turn Off the Empathic Response

You may try your best to elicit an empathic response from your doctor, but there may be times when you do not succeed. Whenever physician–patient communication begins to break down, the physician's empathic response may be the first casualty. A physician who feels ill used will rarely respond sensitively to the patient.

Here is the case of Janice, a young mother who is in despair over her baby's persistent rash. Although she does attempt to express her distress, she remains ineffective. She has gone to other consultants and followed their instructions, but feels that no one has been able to help her. This physician gives her very little opportunity to expand on her concerns. In the last three days, the rash has spread and gotten worse, and neither she nor her baby has had any sleep. She is literally begging for help.

DOCTOR: *How long has this been going on?*

JANICE: *A year.*

DOCTOR: *M-hm.*

JANICE: *Ever since I got back from overseas.*

DOCTOR: *M-hm.*

JANICE: *And uh . . . I just can't, uh . . . I can't . . . I can't stand it any-more. I have just . . . it's getting to the point where I'm going to have a nervous breakdown!*

Although she has told him that she can't take it anymore and she is obviously in great distress, she gets no response to her feeling.

DOCTOR: *M-hm. Well, come on. Lay him on the table. I want to take a look at this.*

(Later)

DOCTOR: *Okay . . . what we need to do is—is get a culture of it.*

JANICE: *Yeah.*

DOCTOR: *And we'll send him to the specialists in dermatology . . . that's what you're doing here.*

JANICE: *Where?*

DOCTOR: (Irritated) *Where's what?*

JANICE: *That's here?* (The dermatologist's office)

DOCTOR: *Sure.*

JANICE: *Oh.*

DOCTOR: *We're not . . . we're not going to send* (short laugh) *you, uh, somewhere else.*

Janice is at the end of her tether and fears that she might get shuttled to yet one more facility. When she simply asks where the specialist is, he literally scoffs at her question. She apologizes:

JANICE: *Oh, well you don't know how . . . how many trips I've been on.*

DOCTOR: *Well, where has he been seen?*

JANICE: *The Naval Hospital in San Diego. Now, they wanted to keep him there.*

DOCTOR: *In the <u>hospital</u>?*

JANICE: *Yeah . . . they took a blood test and took a urinalysis on him.*

DOCTOR: *M-hm.*

JANICE: *And they wanted to take him because he had it for so long and I was . . . and I was giving him . . . .*

DOCTOR: *M-hm.*

JANICE: *. . . you know, excellent treatment, so when I came to Los Angeles here, I said, well . . . it could . . . if it continues, I could have him admitted to the hospital in—*

DOCTOR: (Interrupts) *Well, first of all, see, we don't admit children for impetigo.*

Janice is frightened because she was told her child definitely needed to be in the hospital. Yet this doctor remains unimpressed by her story. He does not respond to her fears, but approaches the problem strictly from a medical establishment point of view. He's looking at the rash and not listening to the mother. She makes one more desperate effort to challenge him:

JANICE: *Well, when there's something like this?*

DOCTOR: *Yes, that's right. He's not a sick boy.*

JANICE: *Yeah, but he's making everybody . . . he's making everybody else sick and I . . .*

DOCTOR: *Well, it's making you nervous and everything.*

The doctor finally acknowledges that she is very upset. For a brief moment, Janice feels understood:

JANICE: (Interrupts) *That's right!*

DOCTOR: *. . . uh, fine, but uh . . . uh, we don't have . . . our . . . we don't have enough beds for the . . . the extremely sick people here and not beds for this sort of thing.*

(Pause)

JANICE: *I don't . . .*

DOCTOR: (Interrupts) *Well . . . well, we don't stick them in the hospital, or we . . . we . . . .*

JANICE: *Even if it was only for two days?*

Here she has again challenged him and he responds by putting her down:

DOCTOR: (Interrupts) *or . . . for who? For him to, uh, sit in the hospital while we wait for our cultures to grow out and uh . . . uh . . . to contaminate everything on the floor with . . . uh . . . staphylococci . . . or for you to just rest?*

JANICE: *I have children at home! No . . . It's not that . . . I'm not getting any rest! I have two children . . . hell. . . . I have a baby and a little girl and he's around them all the time and they can't understand when I tell them "well . . . don't play with him" . . . the baby goes . . . they can't understand that!*

DOCTOR: *M-hm.*

JANICE: *I can't watch. . . . I keep telling them . . . I kept cutting his fingernails . . . I keep . . . you know, don't scratch.*

DOCTOR: *M-hm.*

JANICE: *I mean . . . I . . . I'm not getting any rest. Don't misunderstand me!*

He responds to Janice as being mostly worried about her own comfort. She then has another emotional outburst:

JANICE: *I can't understand why he can't be admitted. I know you have children here maybe that . . . uh . . . have trouble with . . . are sick, but this . . . this, to me, is sickness.*

DOCTOR: *Sure it's a sickness. It's like . . . . We're admitting meningitis . . . people, uh—*

JANICE: (Interrupts) *I understand that—*

DOCTOR: *And this boy has had this for a year!*

JANICE: *I know it and I think it's been too long.*

DOCTOR: *And it's a skin problem . . .*

JANICE: *Don't you think I know that?*

DOCTOR: *. . . and he's perfectly . . . other than the skin disease, he's a healthy boy.*

JANICE: *He's a healthy boy. I know that.*

DOCTOR: *And we . . . so we don't admit people like that in the hospital here.*

JANICE: (Sighs)

Janice has given up for the moment.

DOCTOR: (Resumes) *Well!*

JANICE: *Well, I think it's pretty silly, myself. You don't understand! It's like a race track [at my home] . . . because . . . <u>look</u> at my son like that! I've been troubled with this stuff for years and it made me mad . . . .* (Beginning to cry) *I'm tired of it!*

Doctor: *All right! I'm offering . . . I'm offering you—uh—as I say, the logical approach, what the medical profession does to handle this thing. We're not a babysitting service!*

The doctor abandons all efforts to really listen and respond to her as a human being. He justifies his behavior as being the logical approach of the medical profession. At this point, Janice breaks into tears. <u>The doctor offers her neither Kleenex or comfort.</u>

JANICE: *I don't need you for it! I've got babysitters . . . my mother babysits . . . my mother-in-law . . . my child has these doggone things on his skin and I have been taking care of him and I just don't . . . and evidently whatever I have done is not doing him any good. And I'm tired of it!*

Janice was still crying when she left his office.

At first glance, the physician in this encounter seems insensitive and ultimately hostile. Why wasn't he more responsive with the distraught mother? One reason, which does not excuse his lack of empathy, might be that physicians have a tendency to dislike encounters with patients who have ongoing illnesses that are not improving. As soon as he hears that this child has had the rash for a year, this doctor began to distance himself. Also, Janice was extremely defensive. She did not clearly indicate that she was willing to work with him. She attacked and defended, attacked and defended, and in the end they were just arguing.

This battle is similar to the kind of dispute that takes place when a marriage is breaking up. A couple contemplating divorce gives up all hope of communicating with each other. When there is an argument, they no longer make an effort to listen to one another or understand each other's feelings. All each one wants to do is win. While one is talking (or shouting), the other is preparing the next line of attack.

It is worth learning from Janice's mistakes. She turned the doctor off right from the beginning by being overly emotional. During the first few exchanges, she focused almost exclusively on her own reactions. Instead of discussing her child's problem, she concentrated on herself: "*I just can't . . . I can't . . . I can't stand it anymore*," threatening to have a nervous breakdown.

At the beginning of an appointment, it is important for the patient to engage the physician with the problem itself. When Janice mentioned her impending nervous breakdown, this physician felt ill used because this was outside of his sphere of professional competence. At this point the encounter began to completely break down and everything slid downhill from there.

She came to the appointment with a fixed agenda to get her child hospitalized. In justifying her argument, she concentrated on her own reactions and her family situation rather than describing her child's illness. Trying to escape the increasingly intense emotional onslaught, the doctor focused his attention entirely on the medical task. Another one of her tactics sure to upset the physician was to quote other authorities when she did not like what he said. She told him what other doctors had said and quickly stressed that they agreed with her point of view. When patients talk about what "the other doctor" said, physicians justifiably think,

If you prefer the solution offered by someone else, then what are you doing here talking to me?

A good thing to remember is that when you indicate to your doctor how highly you value other opinions, you may be coming across as threatening, and this will undermine the relationship. In this case, Janice gave the implicit message that she did not trust this doctor, but was trying to persuade him with what others had said.

Instead of asking for help, she virtually gave the doctor an assignment: *"Hospitalize my child!"* that immediately put him on the defensive. When the doctor lost his cool and became angry, she became more defensive and tried to bargain with him, *"Could you put him in for two days?"* Again, she was telling him what to do. Doctor and patient engaged in a continuing battle and never found common ground. Had she let the doctor know

"I need help. I don't know what to do for this child at home. I would like to keep him at home, I have plenty of people to help me, but I have tried everything I know and now I think maybe he needs to be in a place where people can take better care,"

things might have turned out differently.

When you visit a physician, do you expect him or her to read your mind and guess your feelings? Patients often believe their doctors will automatically know how they are feeling and what they need. Although medical information is routine to physicians, it can trigger stronger anxieties in patients than doctors often anticipate. A patient, Cathy, went to her doctor for her yearly gynecological checkup and a few days later got a call from his office informing her,

"Dr. X. would like to see you as soon as possible. Your Pap smear came back a number 4."

She went in immediately, endured a painful biopsy procedure, and during a follow-up appointment, Dr. X told her that she had cervical dysplasia, a precancerous condition that required her to go into the hospital for outpatient surgery. He explained that the procedure would be routine and simple—he would remove the precancerous cells with a laser beam. In her mid-twenties and having been healthy all her life, Cathy found the word "precancerous" devastating. When she left her doctor's office, she started crying. She got into her car and was barely able to get home. She called her husband Roger at his office and was so upset that she could hardly explain what had happened. Alarmed, her husband called the doctor and told him that his wife was crying uncontrollably. The doctor then called Cathy at home:

> DOCTOR: *Roger called me and told me that you are upset.*
>
> CATHY: *Yeah, well, you said I have cancer.*
>
> DOCTOR: (Alarmed) *I did <u>not</u> tell you that you have cancer. I told you that you have a form of a <u>precancerous</u> condition. You do <u>not</u> have cancer.*
>
> CATHY: *I don't have cancer?*
>
> DOCTOR: *No, you don't have cancer. I explained to you that precancer is not cancer. The cells are precancerous, that's not the same as cancer. You'll go into the hospital next week, I'll do the laser procedure to remove the abnormal cells, and you'll be fine.*
>
> CATHY: *I will?*
>
> DOCTOR: *Yes.*
>
> CATHY: *Yes . . . okay . . . .*
>
> DOCTOR: *Why didn't you tell me you were this upset when you were here?*
>
> CATHY: *I don't know . . . .*

Before you decide that your doctor's responses do not meet your needs, you should try your best to make your feelings known. It is up to us as patients to make sure that our doctors do understand:

> *"I know you have already explained it to me, but I was too upset to really understand. Please explain it again.*
>   *"I'm really apprehensive about the surgery even though you say it's just a simple outpatient procedure. Actually, I'm afraid of the whole thing."*

If your doctor does not respond, then you should insist:

"I don't think you're aware of how upsetting this is to me, . . ."

and then explain how it is affecting you.

While doctors so frequently get blamed for being poor communicators, patients also have difficulty expressing themselves and often expect their doctors to magically guess their needs. It's similar to the kind of situation that happens in some marriages when a wife who is a working professional as well as the one who cooks the evening meals has been hoping to be taken out for dinner. Here she has worked all week, prepared suppers, and she becomes disappointed because it doesn't occur to her husband to give her a break by suggesting they go out for dinner. She finally gets angry and her husband, puzzled, asks why she is so upset. She says,

"Well, I've been cooking dinner all week in addition to my job and I'm tired!"

He replies,

"Oh darling, do you want to go out to dinner, I didn't know! Let's make a reservation right away."

By then it is too late. His invitation no longer counts because she had to suggest it. She wants him to have been sensitive enough to guess it and then do something about it on his own.

Reflect on what you really want and what is acceptable to you. If your doctor responds empathically by opening up and talking to you about your concerns, then you have successfully broken the silence. When your doctor is not responsive, it may be that you haven't expressed yourself in a way that allowed the doctor to understand. And when patients don't reach out, even the most highly motivated doctors may get discouraged and give up. I gave a lecture to the staff of a large county hospital in Geneva this past summer and, after I had finished, a young doctor came up to me and asked,

"What do you do when you keep trying to reach out to a patient and it never works? I have this one patient who I've had real trouble with in the last several visits. I've tried to establish a warm relationship, I've

tried to get to know her, and I just can't get across to her. She doesn't respond to me."

He was extremely frustrated in his effort to be a humane physician.

Remember that physicians are not the same with different patients, different problems, and on different days. Are you looking for technical expertise? Do you want a doctor who is interested in the relationship and goes out of his or her way to communicate? Does your doctor respond to your feelings? Have you ever been offended by your doctor's attitude? One patient went to a clinic for care and, when she began expressing some of her concerns, was actually told by a physician,

"This is a one-problem clinic; we really don't have time for more."

None of us are one-problem patients! If you are anxious and ask your doctor for help, but he or she lets you down, then perhaps your best move would be to request a referral to someone who is willing to spend some time with you. Another alternative is to bide your time and see if you can negotiate a change in the relationship. How long have you been going to this doctor? Have you really tried to foster a good relationship? If both of you make an effort, the relationship could change for the better.

As I think about what seems reasonable for patients to expect, I consider the relationships I have with my own doctors and realize that I would like them to *understand* my feelings and accept them, although they cannot necessarily share them. And always, as patients, we need to hold up our end of the communication process and maintain an awareness that we too have a responsibility. Instead of quietly accepting what our doctors say or do not say and then going home and complaining to our family and friends, we need to speak up.

HOW DO DOCTORS
GET THAT WAY?

The Conspiracy of Silence

If the emotional dilemmas encountered by medical students in training are disregarded or dealt with only incidentally or accidentally, the students will stumble in their desperation into the maladaptive roles seen all around us in graduate physicians. The students will meet these issues by transmuting their patients into abstractions, which offer neither the pain nor the gratification of human intimacy. They will take refuge from human responsibility in obsessive attention to detail.

LOREN STEPHENS, M.D.

This statement was made by a physician who felt that, during his education and early professional career, he had had insufficient help in dealing with his own suffering and vulnerability. This is not a unique experience; most students, young physicians, and practicing physicians have had little help with these problems. Feelings are not acknowledged in the course of traditional medical education. The reluctance on the part of practitioners and medical educators to discuss patients' feelings and especially their own feelings has been referred to as a "conspiracy of silence."

How do doctors become the seemingly "feelingless," matter-of-fact kinds of physicians whom patients complain about? Are they insensitive people to begin with? Probably not, because we all know that every human being has the potential for feeling empathy. In a daycare center, when one toddler starts to cry, the others are sure to join in. There has been much speculation about the genesis of empathy in human beings and in animals. Every pet owner knows that when the master is upset, the faithful cat or dog will come over and try to offer comfort. In one experiment, two small monkeys were placed in a situation where only one would be exposed to a painful stimulus at a time.[1] They could see each other's faces on a television monitor. It turned out that when one monkey was experiencing pain and showed distress in its face, the other one demonstrated empathy by pushing a lever that stopped the painful stimulus.

Is it something that happens in doctors' training? Some explanations for the apparent absence of responsiveness lie in the traditions of medical education. How does it all begin? To study medicine and be successful, you have to excel in many courses, do well on exams, and be aggressive and competitive to get ahead. You must devote all your energy to perform at the highest level. You receive little encouragement to participate in anything other than the requisite hard-core science classes, and you are expected to get nothing lower than A's. Medical students are so terribly busy that they have no free time and very little private life. This keeps them from participating in many of the normal social interactions that would allow them to assume an adult role in society. They are given insufficient opportunity to develop their personalities. While many of their friends and acquaintances are entering adult society—getting married, having children, buying houses and cars—their lives are becoming increasingly impoverished. They lose themselves as human beings. Those extra five, six, seven years of training are like a delayed adolescence. They become so enmeshed in their studies that they are cut off from music, art, reading, and they work so hard that they are too tired to participate in normal activities. Even the very basic self-maintenance errands that we all take for granted like going to the grocery store or getting a haircut become special events.

In one of our support groups, an intern told me about finally having the opportunity to visit a grocery store after a month on call at the hospital:

"I really enjoyed shopping around, looking at mushrooms, and thinking about what I was going to make. But when I got in the checkout line, this perfect stranger turned around to me and said, 'You really look tired.' A perfect stranger in the Safeway telling me how tired I was!"

Another intern described getting a haircut after working all night:

"I saw the barbershop and said to myself, 'I'll feel better if I get a haircut.' So I go in and I'm getting the haircut, sleeping the whole time, I had no idea what the guy was doing to my hair. He finally looked at me and said, 'You look pretty tired, what do you do?' I said, 'Oh, I was working last night.' I didn't tell him what I did. He asked, 'How old are you?' So I said, 'How old do you think I am?' And, honest to God, without a smile on his face he said thirty-seven."

The intern was actually more than ten years younger.

The Start of Dehumanization

Until very recently in most medical schools, the first human "patient" a medical student encountered was almost always a cadaver. Most courses in gross anatomy schedule an early exercise that consists of dissecting a human being, one of the first rites of passage for doctors-to-be. At this point in their education, these students have no more preparation for the experience than you do. The encounter is dreaded by students; many have never even seen a dead person, much less touched one. When the time arrives, they are faced with actually having to look at, touch, and cut the body. Most students are frightened and repelled. Cadavers smell strongly of formaldehyde, come wrapped in gauze, and must be doused with fluids regularly so that they don't dry out. While many students are able to overcome their revulsion, others are tempted to take flight and in some instances students have even fainted.

The dissection involves breaking a lot of deeply ingrained taboos in not only touching but cutting parts of the body that are usually held to be private and untouchable—the genitals and the internal organs. Students often cope with the experience by treating their cadaver with black humor—they name it, talk about it in jest, and speculate what sort of life the person might have led. During the course of the dissection, they gradually work on more and more of the body until they finally uncover the head. It is usually left until last because it is complicated and involves the intricate details of the central nervous system, which makes it one of the most difficult dissections. They frequently find this last experience emotionally wrenching because they are finally forced to see the face and become aware that their cadaver was indeed someone. Although they have worked on the rest of the body for months, they have to accept that the human being they are dissecting once had an identity and a personality.

In the course of the first two years of medical study, students concentrate on anatomy, chemistry, physiology, and pathology. They are required to absorb a tremendous amount of scientific information that does not seem relevant to actual medical practice. More often than not, it appears to them that the basic reasons for which they chose to study medicine have been pushed aside. Students ask themselves,

"What am I doing here? I wanted to be a doctor and help sick people; I don't see how this is getting me there."

Then, finally, when third-year students have their first intense encounter with real patients, they are faced with sickness and death in very large doses. Overwhelmed, one of the students commented,

"I didn't realize when I chose to study medicine that I was going to spend the rest of my life with sick people!"

They begin to feel vulnerable and become increasingly aware that they themselves could become sick or even die. You can't deal with sick people without becoming acutely aware that you also could become very sick. And encountering dying patients makes them reflect on their own mortality. Students often get the same symptoms as their patients, a phenomenon referred to as "medical student's disease." When they start learning about tuberculosis, for example, it isn't long before they think they have it. One third-year medical student commented that he had to reassure himself and distance himself from the patients by emphasizing,

> "*This patient is older, he's not like me . . . . This patient is a female, I know I won't develop her disease . . . . This patient is poor, he's not like me.*"

As they go through their studies, students' inner conflicts with facing illness and death become more and more acute. Their role models, the attending physicians, often behave toward them (and their patients!) in ways that are not very human. All too often, attending physicians do not deal with emotional issues and students are thus left to struggle with them on their own. Knowledge of anatomy and technical skills are emphasized exclusively. They are to focus on the task, make the right diagnosis, perform the appropriate technical procedures. They are left alone in their anguish.

In the following interview, a medical student discusses how, in the beginning of his training, he tried to "feel as much as I could feel" only to find out that that did not work:

> "*I've had some, uh, really very mercurial changes between sort of walking on to the ward at the beginning of this year, you know really kind of wanting to embrace everything, and be receptive to whatever kind of input I get. I really did. And to try to feel as much as I could feel . . . I saw a lot of frightening and painful things . . . and discovered for the first time something that I'd heard but not really believed and that was that, at County Hospital anyway, it was just so heavy and so bad . . . you're not effective by being truly empathic. I went through a period of trying to protect myself emotionally by reacting primarily in an intellectual fashion and sort of, in a sense, holding off from my patients, and that didn't work either. For me or the patients. It was sort of like, it was a very subtle thing, setting your 'empathostat.'*"

Another student laughed:

> "*Your empathostat?*"

Students are taught to think of the patient as a problem to solve, not as a human being. In this next interview, a physician told of an experience he had as a medical student when he realized that the pressure to always be right outweighed his concern for his patient:

> "As a medical student, I had a guy who had tuberculosis, and at first when he came in, I thought it was a carcinoma with bone metastases and I had X rays of his bones done. I remember looking at the X rays and being really disappointed because there were no metastases . . . my diagnosis was wrong . . . .
>
> "And then, right after that, about two days later, I realized how disappointed I had been . . . I thought—'You are really perverted . . . . All your training has been so screwed up that you're thinking more of your diagnosis than the patient.'"

Traditionally, medical trainees who show too much sensitivity have been looked down on as being "weak." One of the goals in the education of physicians is to "professionalize" them, to toughen them up so that they will not be too sensitive. They learn to approach patients and their diseases in a professional rather than a personal, subjective manner. In this next interview, a medical student discusses the first days of training in a hospital, the intern who was his role model, and when he began to realize that he was becoming what was considered a "good" doctor:

> "I remember my first couple of days at the hospital. I had a really, really boorish and crass intern, just an incredibly callous, haughty, individual who really had no business in medicine. I'm not naive about people to begin with, and none of us are, it wasn't like we were so vastly impressionable that this person was going to mold us for the future . . . . He was the first intern I was going to follow around, he was kind of a model, and it was frightening to me.
>
> "There were certain hang-ups I was going through at the time, things like inflicting pain . . . . I would get upset, for example, if I was trying to take arterial blood out of somebody's wrist, and the needle goes deep enough that it hits the bone and they would scream . . . . I would get upset . . . and the intern would scoff at me about that. That's

extreme, but what I began to eventually realize as I became more familiar with this is that there are pressures [in the system] not to be moved by those kinds of feelings, not to experience those things.

"If the intern had said, 'That must be hard for you . . . ,' we would have discussed the reasons why it was a difficult procedure for me. But what was encouraged was a pseudo-bravery that can only be fostered by self-imposed callousness.

"I eventually learned the trade pretty well, and, as I learned, I became more efficient at it. As I became more efficient, I began to get more praise. I was regarded as a better doctor because I could go in and stick that needle in and it wouldn't hit bone anymore. I really began to wonder, 'Well, how am I accepting myself? What's the basis for my faith in myself?'

"When I first came in here, I saw all kinds of really blatant behavior. I saw it institutionalized to a point where those were standard behaviors. But my whole feeling about being taught and being encouraged to have inadequate and maladaptive defenses is really important . . . I see people around who have not dealt with these issues any better than I have. They either repress it, or they dissociate it, and then when something happens and the balance is tipped and they just can't repress, then they have an anxiety attack."

These quotations were part of a videotape we showed during a seminar for a well-known medical society at the Los Angeles Biltmore Hotel. It was so disastrous that we have traditionally referred to it as the "Biltmore Bomb." In the audience were physicians with established practices who were members of the "silent generation"—that is, they respected the conspiracy of silence about doctors' feelings. These doctors never talk about their own emotions or those of their patients; when they gather in doctors' lounges, hospital cafeterias, or surgeons' waiting areas, their conversations are about neutral subjects like new technology and golf scores. My seminar dealt with the anxieties and concerns of young people entering the medical profession. It initially elicited very little response from the audience, but when they saw the videotape we had produced, in which students bitterly expressed their anger and distress about how they had been trained into *not* feeling, the audience came to life. One physician interjected,

*"All of us went through medical training, we weren't allowed to com-
plain, and here we are! We turned out all right!"*

The audience had no sympathy for these medical students and were absolutely horrified as they watched them expressing their anguish and baring
their souls before the camera. They insisted that such behavior was totally
inappropriate, that the subjects in the video were "weaklings," and that they
should never have been selected for medical school. A physician commented angrily,

*"These students are neurotic and emotionally imbalanced! They just
want to roll around in their own muck."*

After Medical School

During internship and residency, trainees continue to confront morbidity,
mortality, and vulnerability, only now the training is even more intense. The
first year of internship is a high-risk time for dehumanization. These are
sleep-deprived, overworked, exhausted doctors who are overwhelmed with
clinical problems. Trainees are suddenly swamped with high numbers of
sick patients, carry a tremendous burden of clinical care, and are under pressure to perform. If you ask most interns what the worst part of their training was, they mostly say that they were overwhelmed by the workload. And
still, just as in the undergraduate years, while there is a great amount of
attention focused on technical skills, there is no reinforcement to maintain
natural human responses. They get no help in dealing with their emotions
and, as a result, they begin to defend themselves against them, eventually
shutting them off. An intern told me,

*"There's no one to help me with my feelings, the faculty does not under-
stand, and the other interns can't help me. They are so busy with their
own problems. There's no one."*

One of the unfortunate features of training is that it traditionally takes
place on hospital wards, which means that these new doctors never get the
opportunity to really get to know patients and their families. They see sick

patients in bed and may never see them dressed or sitting upright They may never meet other family members or know anything about the patient's outside life. Although they are learning about their patients' diseases, they have no opportunity to get gratification from their patients as human beings. They are under high pressure to perform and, when they are evaluated, it is on the basis of their technical skills and knowledge rather than their humanity.

When graduate trainees begin to seriously participate in patient care, it causes them to realize that it is they who are now responsible. They really are on the spot. One intern revealed an experience in which he became acutely aware of the extent of his responsibility even in doing a simple test.[2] He described how on his first night on "Admitting," a young girl came in at 4 A.M. suffering from what appeared to be a drug overdose. He performed a lumbar puncture to check for the possibility of meningitis, and had to make a special Gram stain from the smear. In the laboratory, he'd done many such stains from other patients he didn't know, but this time it was different. He told me,

> "It acutely came to my mind . . . that whatever I said or wrote down on the chart was going to be accepted by the resident, by the staff people who came around, and by everyone else. Probably no one would double-check me, and, if I were wrong, there would be dire consequences. And I repeated that Gram stain seven times at 4 A.M. in the morning because I was scared about the responsibility I had."

Interns become preoccupied with diagnosis, treatment, and life-threatening illnesses. When you try to engage them on personal issues, they are so anxious that they can't stop thinking such things as,

> What if I don't make the correct diagnosis? What's going to happen if I am the one in the emergency room and a patient stops breathing? What if I have to resuscitate somebody?

These fears are realistic. And, as patients, there is no question that we do want to be confident that they know how to perform those tasks expertly. But when these young doctors are solely concerned with the technical end of medical care, as their role models strongly encourage and reinforce, almost no emphasis is given to the human aspects of medicine.

In our intern support groups, we learned that many young physicians felt that no one seemed to be aware of the extent to which they were suffering. Here is where the "conspiracy of silence" begins to manifest itself. Trainees feel so brutalized that when they are with patients, they have little left to give. Their own suffering is neither recognized nor discussed, and becomes so acute that it is very hard for them to be empathetic with patients.

Another factor contributing to their dehumanization and lack of responsiveness to patients is that they are simply overwhelmed by their workload. Everything else goes by the wayside. They become so aware of their own fatigue and distress that they are no longer open to the experiences of their patients. Sleep deprivation does change a person's ability to function; it also takes away much of your sensitivity and responsiveness. The philosophy underlying medical education is much like that used in training soldiers—unless they learn to function under stress, they will not be able to work successfully under stress in the battlefield. And so for medical trainees, it is indeed a trial by hard knocks much like combat training. They are constantly fatigued. Interns reach a state of mind where if, for instance, a patient says,

"You know, I'm so tired lately . . . ."

the intern automatically thinks,

You say __you're__ tired? I'm the one who's been up all night.

Young doctors who don't have the chance to develop into complete mature human beings may become flawed. To react as one human being to another is what empathy is all about, and this very basic human response becomes nearly impossible. An intern who had recently completed his first year described the pressure he was under and admitted bitterly,

"I don't look forward to seeing patients anymore, I just dread having to see anybody. The internship has done this to me. I didn't used to be this way."

In an interview, one intern discussed how the huge numbers of admissions had taken away her sympathy and empathy for patients:

> *"It bothers me a little bit . . . these people, even though we think it's minor illness and everything, we're still the major contact at the hospital for them and we have so little sympathy and empathy to give . . . . Our sympathy and empathy just isn't there . . . . It doesn't seem very human. That's what makes our institutions inhuman. It is the pressure of time and workload that I think creates that. I think we all like to be busy and get interesting admissions, but we don't like to be pushed to the point where we have no sympathy for anybody."*

Here an intern tells the interviewer that she has no time to talk with patients and that when she does, it "sets her back."

> *"Well, when you're carrying thirteen, fifteen patients, your interaction with patients and their families becomes minimal at best. I think there are certain times when you can spend a little more time talking to patients, but I haven't found it to be that often. And when you do, it just sets you back. There's a limit on what you can do. Is it more important to look at his chest X ray or talk to the family? And you're the intern, you're the one who is supposed to look at the chest X ray."*

This next intern is angry because he has been stretched beyond his limit. He no longer has sympathy for his patients and even feels animosity toward some of them.

> *"I get angry in the emergency room. That's the one place where I don't have sympathy or empathy anymore, when I go to the ER. If I go into a room and we have a fat baby on the bed and the complaint is that the baby won't eat, I am livid. If it's a busy day, I'm just so mad and I go around mad all day down there because it's a Saturday and we're swamped and we're backed up four hours. Ninety percent of the patients are going to make me so mad . . . the typical complaint that comes in there now I have no patience for. Last July or August I did."*

Interns believe that they have to be perfect—anything less means that they are not living up to their own expectations. One of the exercises I found very helpful in my support groups with trainees was to have them make a list of attributes they think are necessary for being a good physician. Their lists are always incredibly long and ambitious. The "good" physician they envision has a level of perfection no human being could possibly attain. Doctors in just about all stages of their careers struggle with these self-expectations on their own and this contributes to their not being as open with themselves, their patients, and their colleagues about their reactions to situations. What this means is that they end up feeling it is unacceptable not to like a patient, to be unhappy to get up in the middle of the night to help a patient, to be lazy, to be wrong. They carry a tremendous burden of guilt because they think they have to do everything perfectly all the time. Consequently, when anything goes wrong, they blame themselves mercilessly. This burden does not end with the role of physician; they are also obliged to neglect their personal lives.

In this next interview, an intern married to a businessman doubly blames herself. When she spends time with her husband and does not study, she feels guilty. When she studies and does not spend time with her husband, she feels guilty.

> "Because I'm married, being a female, there are certain expectations with my husband's job. Other wives go along for certain functions and I'm just not that available.
>
> "I had such tremendous guilt feelings this year when I wasn't able to be with him. I was either at the hospital or asleep.
>
> And if I did have any time, I didn't use it to read, which I felt tremendously guilty about because I felt that I needed to do some reading and I had virtually done zero—it came down to either spending the time with my husband or doing some reading. If I was with him, I felt guilty about not doing the reading; if I was doing the reading, I felt guilty about not being with him."

The stress of training is overwhelming not only for the weaker trainees. The following account was given by an intern who was highly regarded by his peers and supervisors and seemed to be functioning exceptionally well.

> "The defects or weaknesses in your personality that you bring with you, you have to handle those under such enormous stress that if you are not

a self-confident person in one way or another, those
lenged all the time because you are here all the time. Y
decision making are much more important than they ⌣
you have to deal with your own problems, whatever they are, .
situations where there is no time out, it's constant everyday, all day,
seven days a week, month after month after month. You don't have a
chance to deal with your own problems, you just have to defensively
survive.

"*It was so stressful, I never thought it would be as stressful as it*
was . . . it just keeps coming, it never stops. You get to the point where
it's 4 o'clock in the morning and it's your one hundredth admitting
night, and I go into the elevator and cry for about fifteen minutes. And
I think, 'Why am I doing this? It's so awful. . . . Why do it? What's the
point? It doesn't seem reasonable.'"

The Impact on Patient Care

So what difference does this all make? How are patients affected and how does it affect physicians in practice? Internship is like a military experience. Soldiers who have been through a war are less sensitive to feelings because they have seen people getting hurt and killed. Similarly, doctors-in-training live in an environment where they see sick and dying people, yet no one cares about their own emotions or their pain. Consequently, when patients complain about their problems, physicians typically focus on the technical details they need to hear and shut out everything else.

Doctors who are viewed by patients as being distant may themselves have been overwhelmed by their own feelings during training. When our feelings become too painful and too powerful, we may "shut the door" to protect ourselves. The trouble is that when you close certain doors consistently, you may never be able to open them again.

To study physician behavior during hospital rounds, a group of attending physicians and their trainees were followed as they interacted with their patients. My research team and I videotaped the encounters on a busy adult ward where curtains were the only separation between the beds. We stopped at a bed and watched as one of the interns began examining a patient. As we observed his procedures, I realized that the patient in the adjacent bed had become violently ill. Although we could not see this other patient, we ost definitely could hear him. When no one came to help him, he began calling, *"Doctor! Nurse! Can't someone help me?"* The intern paid no attention and continued to focus on his own patient. The attending physician supervising him also completely ignored the cries for help. When I interviewed the intern afterwards, I asked, *"Were you troubled at all by the patient in the next bed? He seemed so uncomfortable and was calling for help."* The intern responded, *"No, I've really gotten much better at that . . . I don't hear things like that anymore."*

Overidentification

Many doctors distance themselves from patients, perhaps to a fault, but there are also risks when physicians become too close. While the issue of overidentifying with patients is overwhelming to the student, it is a problem some physicians continue to struggle with throughout their medical careers. If a trainee does not learn to deal with overidentification, it will probably resurface later in practice. This physician may be the kind of doctor who suffers too much and, as a result, patient care also suffers. Sometimes a patient's condition relates to a personal experience the physician has had. Perhaps a patient reminds the physician of a close friend or family member.

I became involved with a case some years ago in which the surgeon's patient reminded him so much of his own son that it influenced the child's health care. This surgeon was taking care of a boy who, in physical appearance and behavior, was strikingly similar to his own son. Because of his feelings for the patient, the surgeon was reluctant to perform the surgery. The child had been found to have a tumor on his foot when he was about six years old and the surgeon had removed it. But it continued to recur and, after many more procedures, it became necessary to perform a mid-calf amputation. A few years later, the boy came back with a painful swelling at the site where the prosthesis attached to his leg. If the child had not reminded him so vividly of his own son and if he had not been so emotionally involved with him, the surgeon would undoubtedly have decided to biopsy the swelling immediately. Instead, he decided to wait and observe because he simply could not accept the idea that the tumor had recurred. Here are excerpts from my talks with the patient, whom I'll call Mark, and the surgeon.

MARK: *There was one operation, between the third grade and fourth, there was one big operation that almost got rid of it [the tumor]. He cut up and around, through between the toes, and clear up the foot, then over near the ankle and he cut off one of the toes and he took the muscles out and he took out a big bone in my foot, then on the bottom, cut along the ball of my foot and then up and over and opened it up . . . he really tore it apart. The foot didn't look like much after that.*

SURGEON: *This boy was a very traumatic experience for me. It originally started out with a little nodule on his foot which was thought to be a neuro-fibroma, but it spread and we did a second and third and a fourth operation, each one becoming more vigorous, taking bones—eventually we did an amputation from the mid-calf. He's now thirteen but he first came to me around age six—so he's been coming to me six going on seven years. We finally amputated him at the mid-calf about three years after our previous operations. Well, it will be three years the twelfth of this November . . . how interesting that I remember the date . . . .*

He came to the office two weeks ago with a swelling behind the knee, where the prosthesis makes a little pressure. It was quite swollen . . . . Now, mind you, I have positive feelings toward this boy. He's thirteen, my son is fourteen, they have blond hair, he's lovely, likable, you can't help but have positive feelings for him. I have an awful lot of feeling for this person, having dealt with him, having mutilated him over the years and so on. So the boy comes into the office and the first thing that comes into my mind is tumor, but it's a totally unacceptable idea to me. I began making excuses—in my own mind I was thinking—"Well, we'll measure it and see him later in a week."

What I was really doing I think was pulling the covers over my head and hoping that it would go away. If we're going to do it next week, it's not going to go away. If I'd seen this boy come in off the street having arrived from New York six days before and he came to me and I had no relationship with him, unquestionably at that time I would have said this needs biopsy immediately. Again my medical decision at that time was not influenced only by what I read in the books, it was influenced by my relationship to that child . . . to mea-

sure it next week. Well, measuring it next week, had I not had any
positive feelings or other feelings for this boy would have been kind
of ridiculous really. It had to be biopsied, but it was an unacceptable
idea to me.

The things that Mark said to me later about the experience showed me that
this thirteen year old was able to perceive that his doctor's emotions were
involved. Mark noticed that, during a visit, his doctor suddenly left the
room, allegedly to get a Coke, but when he returned Mark could tell that
he was very upset. He was impressed to see his doctor's emotional reaction to him in that situation. He was aware of the impact of his own personality:

MARK: *I see some kids that have real bad personalities, I can just see why*
         they picked me to have this instead of them, because if they had it,
         they would be sunk.

DOCTOR: *I have a son who looks like Mark, he's blond and his hair*
         comes out like this, you know, they like it long and it comes out kind
         of funny. Where I live, our kids are in bands, they have good bands,
         they do the drum major bit, and my son is a junior-high boy who is
         very like Mark in appearance. He plays in the band, but he is always
         practicing in the backyard. It's a big thing to be a drum major . . . .
         When I was getting ready to operate on Mark, I went over to see my
         son perform one time and it was just too much. Ordinarily, I feel
         very proud of him . . . and there are all sorts of things going through
         my mind . . . and it touches me and breaks me up . . . . And when I
         see him marching and I know that I have to take a boy's leg off . . .
         it was very hard to watch those kids.

         *My vacation had been scheduled the week before I **had** to*
         amputate Mark's leg. During the week, when I was working in the
         yard, I could get pretty far away from Mark. I used to always mow
         the lawn by hand but I had recently bought a power mower and I
         was using it. When you stop it to empty the grass basket, the blades
         still go around. At the time, I was miles and miles and miles away
         from Mark, I don't mean in distance but in thought. I stopped to
         empty the grass catcher and the blades were still going around. It

was a little too soon to empty it because it wasn't full but the grass was falling out. I put my hands down very carefully to push the grass out of the way so it wouldn't fall out of the basket, and I said to myself, "Boy that thing really goes around awfully fast, you have to be mighty careful lest you catch your hands in there . . . and then I won't have to operate on Mark." It came to me like that—I saw my hands in bandages and it meant "I don't have to do the operation."

In retrospect, this surgeon was able to show remarkable sensitivity and insight in how his own reactions influenced the care of his patient. In caring for this patient over the years, he had failed to maintain a completely professional attitude. He cared *too* much. He thought of his patient from the point of view of a father, rather than from that of a physician. In one of our work-study groups, he later mentioned that, earlier in his career, he had had a tendency to, as he put it, "sit on my emotions," suppressing them, not taking them into account. But as he gained more experience, he realized that he could not permanently repress them.

While overidentification can have a negative effect on the doctor–patient relationship, if physicians cut themselves off from their patients, medical care will be affected. If a physician's emotional defenses prevent him or her from responding sensitively, then the physician cheats the patient.

An intern consulted me about a little girl she was seeing in the urgent care clinic who had been brought in by her father. The child had vague symptoms—a slight fever with a cough and mild aches and pains that you expect with flu-like illnesses. Neither I nor the intern was this patient's regular physician; the girl was being seen as an "acute visit." The intern told me that when she examined the child, she found nothing wrong and tried, without success, to reassure the father. But he kept insisting, "*She had a 99.5 fever again last night and her legs ache.*" The intern repeatedly tried to explain that the examination had been normal and that her symptoms were due to a cold, but the father still would not accept it. Impatient and becoming annoyed with the patient's father, the intern realized she was getting nowhere and could not get a handle on the situation.

I accompanied her into the examination room and, after the proper introductions, began to ask the father some questions about himself and his family. When I inquired about other children, everything started to clear up. He explained that he had another daughter who was upstairs in the hospital with leukemia. Her illness had begun with slight fevers and diffuse aches, symptoms much like those we were seeing in this patient. His great concern, of course, was that she might have the same illness. The intern had done an adequate technical job, but she had not achieved sufficient communication with the father. She had not reached out enough to empathize with him or to respond properly to the father's anxiety. She had done everything she had been taught to do: she had taken a medical history, done a thorough physical, and made sure that it was nothing serious. But she had failed to realize the full potential that a physician has for helping patients. The father needed help, needed to trust his doctor, but he had been shortchanged. The intern had not identified with him, she had shut him out, and had reacted negatively because his behavior had been annoying to her. It was her job to explore the reasons for his anxiety and had she spent a few moments doing so, there would have been a better outcome.

This is a common problem. When physicians respond to patients exclusively as technicians interested only in scientific aspects, they are not able to achieve a complete therapeutic alliance. These relationships falter, because patients lack trust and feel discouraged. And having invested time and money for the appointment, they also feel cheated and misunderstood. Some may later delay seeking medical care when it is necessary. Others end up making their own diagnoses and treatments, using self-prescribed over-the-counter medications. And some embark on expensive and often fruitless doctor-shopping forays.

If you, as a patient, find that your doctor either does not respond to you or reacts in an unexpected way, there may be reasons. Perhaps you struck a nerve. You may have triggered an issue that is emotionally disturbing or one that your doctor has difficulty handling. He may never have been taught the skills that would help him respond appropriately. As a result, he is ill at ease and uncomfortable.

Throughout medical education, priority is given to the technical and scientific, while an insufficient emphasis is placed on the human aspects of care. A continuing problem is that the interactions of medical students and interns with their patients are rarely evaluated. In fact, quite a few programs allow a young doctor to go through three or four years of training without ever being observed while talking with or examining patients. They are overly busy doing things *to* patients, things that are very often painful, and they don't have enough time to listen, interact, or get to know the patients as people. The faculty evaluates how the new physician-in-training presents a case on rounds, whether she knows the literature, and whether she has missed anything.

Although in an ideal world, a young physician should strive to be both sensitive and competent, in reality, students are led to believe that the subjects they are graded and evaluated on are more important than how a patient feels. Success and failure are determined, after all, by test scores and formal evaluations. As a result, medical students and young physicians struggle on their own with some of the most existential and basic emotional issues. And so when physicians are disturbed by certain issues, they either deny them or become overinvolved. They may not have been encouraged to achieve sufficient insight into their own feelings and responses during their education. Their problems are then carried over and can only intensify during their subsequent careers. They remain unable to process these emotional issues, which leaves them frustrated and often leaves their patients disappointed.

Because insufficient attention is given to physicians' emotions during education, we see both types of maladaptive reactions: the doctor who does not care and the doctor who cares too much. The feeling is trained *out* of them and nothing is trained back *into* them that can help them handle the circumstances involved in everyday interactions in patients. These issues have traditionally been swept under the carpet.

What hope is there that things will improve? In recent years, the patient community, both individuals and groups, have confronted medical educators and professionals and have had a definite impact. Fortunately, there are now impressive efforts to reorganize medical education in such a way that an appropriate priority is given to the psychosocial and emotional aspects of medical education and patient care. At one time, entering medical students were a homogeneous group of young, inexperienced candidates, yet we are now seeing more mature individuals with diversified backgrounds electing to practice medicine. In addition, the early years of medical education are being changed to include experiences with authentic, living patients. There are seminars and group discussions dealing with students' feelings and those of their patients. Curricula covering the art of communicating with patients are being introduced and developed. Medical education at all levels is gradually being refocused so that, although the technical and scientific aspects of training are respected, they are no longer exclusively emphasized. This reemphasis in medical education should result in increased responsiveness on the part of physicians that will make it easier for us, as patients, to communicate with them not only on a technical level but also on a human one. But this does not take *us* off the hook. We still must take more responsibility for our own health care.

DO I HAVE TO GO
TO THE DOCTOR?

▼
▼

Am I Really Sick?

How can you tell when you're sick?

"That's easy," one person responded, *"either you are sick or you are well."* But that's not necessarily true. Everyone reacts differently, and there are no standards as to where the dividing line is. What about you? Are you healthy? Do you get sick a lot? The definition depends on the person who is experiencing the symptoms and what his or her perceptions are. There are young people just bristling with good health who exercise hours every day, eat what they consider a healthy diet, and haven't missed a day of work for a year or two. At the other end of the spectrum are those who consider themselves healthy, but who have learned to modify their levels of aspiration. When asked about their health, they may give a positive response at first, *"I'm doing very well,"* but then continue with some modifications:

"Very well considering there aren't many people of my age who are able to do as well as I am. I still work in my yard everyday."

Do you ever find yourself unconsciously putting yourself down for being "sickly"? Have you ever been contemptuous of others who are not well because you yourself are so very healthy? How often have you heard someone described as

"Oh, you know John, he's always sick."

It's prevalent for people to speak of those who get sick a lot with minor illnesses almost as if they are a nuisance to the world:

"You know him, every time we plan something together, he can't come. I heard that even as a child he was always sick."

The idea of being sick is much more subjective than people realize. Most of us have had days when we wake up in the morning, leap out of bed, and really feel wonderful. *"It's a good day, I'm feeling great!"* You have a sense of positive health and well-being. But there are occasions when it is difficult to demarcate the degree of not feeling well which then makes it difficult to decide whether or not you are "sick." There are people to whom it is so important to get to work that, for them to consider themselves really ill, it would take much more than it might for someone whose only obligation that day is to play a round of golf.

Doctors also have a hard time recognizing that they are sick. They are so used to helping other people that it is especially difficult for them to admit that they themselves are sick. When they are, they feel that they should know what's the matter and what to do. Admitting that they need someone else to help is tough.

The well-known sociologist Talcott Parsons first distinguished between having an illness and actually "playing the sick role," a phrase he coined.[1] His definition includes: "a generalized disturbance of the capacity of the individual for normally expected task or role performance . . . beyond his capacity to overcome . . . he can not be held responsible . . . . Illness is interpreted as a legitimate basis for the exemption of the sick individual . . . from his normal role and task obligations."

What does the sick role involve for you? It means that you accept that you are now a patient and allow your behavior to be guided by that. You give up many of your responsibilities, are no longer able to perform at your usual level, and do not expect to engage in your normal physical activities. It isn't that you are unwilling, you are actually unable to perform your daily routines and do not have to feel guilty about it.

Some people are ashamed to admit that they are ill. They are the ones who go to work even though they have fever, chills, and a hacking cough—and may not be very welcome there because of the contagious nature of their symptoms. Then when they finally do go to the doctor, they are diffident and tend to understate their symptoms. Accident-prone people sometimes get so embarrassed about their repeated injuries that they hesitate to go for help. One patient told me:

> *"I don't dare go back to the same emergency room anymore. I cut my finger twice and once I went in with a broken toe. I was embarrassed because I had been there before. I thought they'd just say, 'You again?' Last time I went to a different doctor, even though it was out of my way."*

On the other end of the spectrum are the people who run to the doctor every time they sneeze. They may be unusually anxious in general, which can turn into anxiety about physical function. They are the ones who almost enjoy giving the gory, dramatic descriptions of their symptoms and are always ready to call in sick at work and cancel other planned activities. Sickness becomes a way of getting special attention from those around them who usually become impatient with them. They become the butt of jokes and are unflatteringly referred to as hypochondriacs. Molière even devoted a comical play to the phenomenon and called it *Le Malade Imaginaire*—the man who imagines he is sick.

There are curious and arbitrary criteria—what we usually call symptoms—that are usually invoked for someone to be considered ill. The most specific of these symptoms and the one often given undue significance is whether or not you have a fever. When there is a measurable elevation of the body temperature, people feel justified in declaring themselves sick. You might notice that people who take a sick day from work or school are quick to report that they had a fever. Excuse notes written to school authorities or employers often mention the level the temperature reached to convince the person at the other end that the individual really was sick. There are patients who are so sick they can hardly move, but unless they have a temperature elevation, they don't feel their illness is legitimate. Few other arguments in everyday life carry as much weight as:

"My temperature went up to 103 last night."

Another symptom that legitimizes being sick is losing your appetite or not having eaten anything for a considerable period of time:

"I haven't had a bite to eat since I got up yesterday morning!"

even though not eating for a couple of days, especially if your fluid intake is adequate, is not a terrible tragedy.

We've all known people who complain about every ache and pain probably because they need a little extra attention:

"Oh, I got a headache last night and this morning it's gone. But last night, it was terrible!"
"My back is so painful. Sometimes it hurts right here, and sometimes it's a little higher up."

Then there are people who, for a particular purpose, consciously pretend to be ill when they know they're not. They belong in a totally different group called malingerers. For instance, there have been quite a few cases of healthy young men who pretended to have all kinds of diseases to avoid military service. Healthy students feign illness in order to postpone a dreaded test, avoid teasing from the school bully, or get out of Phys-Ed. And all doctors know perfectly healthy patients who ask for notes excusing them from work for a day or two.

In reality, if one were to do a head count, more people minimize or deny physical illness than there are those who exaggerate symptoms. Yet, the kinds of tests that we put ourselves through and that other people put us through to establish that we are indeed ill almost makes it seem that we are assumed guilty of malingering until we are proven innocent.

There are anxieties and psychological causes for minimizing physical symptoms. Individuals who fear that they are facing serious illness tend to disregard their symptoms. Cancer or another threatening disease is too much for some to even contemplate, and it therefore inspires overwhelming fear and denial. There are many men in middle age or beyond who begin to have difficulty with urination. They are all too ready to attribute this simply to the fact that they are getting on in age. In reality, this symptom may be due to cancer of the prostate. Unfortunately, by denying that there is anything to see a doctor about, such patients may allow the cancer to reach an advanced stage when successful treatment is less likely. By the same token, for fear that they might have cancer of the breast, some women pay no attention when they become aware of a lump, assuming that it is related to their menstrual cycles.

Even just recognizing that you are ill causes anxiety and is a blow to the ego. With many minor illnesses, people try to cope—

"Well, I'll just take it easy and rest, I'll eat right, and take lots of vitamin C."

Even though they know that they are ill, they make the decision to battle the illness on their own. Yet there is quite a distance between defining yourself as being sick and making the decision to actually consult a doctor.

It's difficult to establish a guideline for when to call the doctor. Patients fear that exaggerating symptoms will cause them to be considered hypochondriacs, but they do not want to ignore or minimize symptoms at the risk of serious consequences. Not consulting a physician may result in a longer illness. Your best approach is to have a continuing relationship with a doctor whom you consider your primary physician. When you establish the relationship, you should begin to explore your doctor's opinions and advice about when you do or do not need to consult him or her. If you are in doubt and don't want to bother the doctor, find someone in the office who can answer your questions about what you are experiencing and whether it is cause for alarm. And of course, at the time of your regular checkup, be prepared to discuss any unusual symptoms you have observed.

In this next interview, Lori could not decide whether what she had was serious enough to make an appointment with her doctor. When she finally made a decision, she found herself in a bind:

"I woke up on Wednesday with a sharp pain in my eyelid. When I looked in the mirror, I couldn't see anything wrong and I thought it

was just something that would go away in a day or two. Well, Wednesday went by and on Thursday, when I woke up, it was red and swollen. I thought, 'Uhhh, I don't feel like going to the doctor . . . ,' I had to go to work, and if I went to the doctor it meant driving all the way over there . . . I'd miss the whole day. Besides, I really didn't feel like going to the doctor and I still hoped it would just go away.

"But on Friday, it was worse. It was very swollen and more painful. So, I decided to call the doctor. . . . I dialed and was dismayed when I got the answering service because it was well after 10 A.M. I asked when the doctor would be coming in and the operator informed me that he was gone for the weekend and wouldn't be back until Monday. For emergencies, there was another doctor I could call . . . . So I said, 'Okay, thank you, no this isn't an emergency' and hung up. I didn't consider a swollen eyelid an emergency. And the other doctor probably had a whole list of other patients who were sicker than I was. I thought, I better not call just for this.

"Then, on Saturday, my eye had really gotten bad and I got more worried. It had been going on for three days. I knew there was nobody who could help unless I went to the emergency room. I imagined myself there with extremely sick people . . . so I thought I would just wait through the weekend. I put on hot compresses and wore a protective eye patch.

"Nothing worked. I got so concerned that I went to a pharmacist at the corner drugstore and asked him what to do. The only thing he could give me were homeopathic eye drops that didn't seem to help . . . but I used them over and over again thinking that eventually it would begin to work. It didn't."

On Monday, Lori finally saw her doctor. If she had been more ready to accept that she needed medical attention, a prompt prescription for an antibiotic might have prevented days of discomfort caused by an eye infection. Like many patients, her problem lay in deciding whether she was sick enough to warrant a visit to the doctor. When you are desperately ill, you don't hesitate to go to the doctor. But other times you end up wondering and the decision becomes harder to make. The next time you find yourself in this dilemma, call your doctor's office for help in making the decision.

The Emergency Room

What kinds of symptoms do you consider an emergency? Why is it that so many illnesses seem to get worse at night and accidents tend to happen on Friday evenings or Saturday mornings? Patients begin to feel very anxious:

"I'm not even sure I can wait till tomorrow . . . and waiting through the whole weekend?"

How do you decide what is an emergency? Do you have to be bleeding? At death's door? Or is the fact that you are not feeling well and have no one else to help you enough justification? It is always hard to decide whether and when to go to the doctor. But determining that you need to go to an emergency room can be even tougher. You have to navigate between two different kinds of risks. If you don't go when you think it might be serious, you risk getting worse and may have to face some undesirable consequences. One patient, Beatrice, cut herself while preparing food in the kitchen:

"I was thinking that I shouldn't bother them [the emergency room] just for a cut finger that's bleeding a lot. And it was my little finger, which made me feel even more ridiculous! And so I put on a Band-Aid and thought I might go to the doctor the next day if I still thought it was necessary. But by the time I went the next day, my doctor told me that he could no longer sew up my cut. So they put the finger in a splint and put me on antibiotics."

If a wound is open and can be contaminated over twenty-four hours or more, it cannot be sutured. Beatrice's convalescence took a lot longer and much of her discomfort and inconvenience could have been prevented if she had promptly gone to the emergency room.

If, on the other hand, you do decide to go to the emergency room but are not absolutely sure it's an "emergency," your risks are a long wait and possibly a negative response from the staff.

So you've made the decision—you're going to the emergency room. What should you expect? You may find yourself in a huge, busy waiting area surrounded by patients with urgent and frightening medical problems. A medical office visit isn't always easy, but a visit to the emergency room is, at best, an eye opener and, at worst, a really grueling experience. There is almost always a wait. You may sit there for a long, long time because there is no appointment system and people who come in after you may actually get taken care of first because they are either sicker or more seriously injured than you are.

One patient, Noreen, took a friend who had stepped on a piece of glass to the emergency room. They waited two hours and finally walked out without seeing a doctor: *"After seeing what was going on there, we decided that our problem wasn't that urgent. I took my friend to her regular doctor the next morning and he removed the piece of glass,"* she said later.

In the emergency room, you're in the midst of the underbelly of medical life—there are all kinds of dramatic, grueling surgical and medical problems. A young woman who came down with a really bad chest cold during the weekend feared that she was developing pneumonia and went to an emergency room. As she sat there waiting, she began to wonder whether she even had a right to be there:

> *"I was sitting there with a woman who'd cut off her fingers with a chain saw while gardening. The nurses came out and told her husband to go home and search for the fingers in the hedge, put them in a plastic bag with ice, and bring them in. Then, only a few minutes later, a guy came in who had just had his front teeth knocked out during a baseball game. There was blood everywhere. A few minutes later they brought in a man in cardiac arrest who wasn't even breathing. Although I knew that I was sick and needed to see a doctor, I did not feel entitled to be there. I felt completely out of place."*

She finally had a chest X ray taken and it turned out that her lungs were clear. At that point, she felt even more foolish and guilty for having even gone there. Yet, on that weekend, when she found herself getting sicker and sicker and developing a hacking cough, it had seemed her only alternative.

Do emergency rooms look down on people who come in with something that's not a big deal? Sometimes. One frustrated doctor said to a patient who came in with a skin problem,

> *"We only take care of really sick patients here."*

Another doctor voiced his frustration,

"If I see one more patient in the middle of the night who has the flu and comes in because she's having trouble sleeping, I'm really going to get mad!"

Emergency physicians rightfully see themselves as being trained for saving lives and resuscitating people. They want to devote their time and effort to what they do best. It's natural, then, for them to begin to resent patients who come in with minor problems.

The patient's point of view is not at all the same as the doctor's. A big difference exists between what medical problems patients consider serious and a doctor's perception. Patients tend to take illness more seriously than doctors. And even doctors don't agree. They have different definitions for seriousness. To some physicians, serious means that you might never get better or perhaps even die. To others, serious means that if it is not treated right away, it is dangerous. So the whole idea of what is serious, what is urgent, and what is an emergency is not as clear as you might think.

While going to an emergency room can be a miserable experience, if you really need the service, it's great that it's there. Much of the unpleasantness for the patient is unavoidable, but there are a few ways to improve the experience. The most important thing is to have a continuing relationship with a primary care physician or internist. You should have a clear understanding of the medical group, the system, or the clinic to which your doctor belongs. If you are a known patient in a medical group, there usually will be someone on call. Then, during your regular checkup, ask about the arrangements for evenings and weekends. Is there an answering service? Are any office personnel available? When the doctor is off call, who covers for her? What kinds of calls are answered by the nurse and which ones does he answer himself? You can usually call your doctor's service on evenings or weekends and receive a call back within an hour or so with advice as to what to do and whether or not you should go to an emergency room. Also ask what emergency rooms the doctor and nurse recommend.

It's becoming more and more important for you as a patient to be as well informed about your own health as possible. So when visiting an emergency room physician who is not aware of your history, you must be your own advocate. Health professionals in emergency facilities or urgent care centers often don't have access to your records and know nothing except what you tell them. Very often, patients with chronic illnesses or complex conditions know more about their disease and treatments than anybody else, including, at times, the physicians whom they consult. Inform them of your condition and your general health:

"I have a heart condition and have been taking X for Y years."

If you are allergic to certain drugs, be certain what they are and make it known to any doctor or other health professionals who might be prescribing for you. If you are taking any medications, either know exactly what they are or bring them with you. For patients with complex health conditions, it's of critical importance to inform the emergency room doctor immediately. If you are a dialysis patient, for example, and have to visit the emergency room for a seemingly unrelated condition such as a sore throat or a bad headache, you need to tell the doctor,

"I am a dialysis patient and I was last dialyzed ____ . Here are the medications I am taking. My doctor's name and telephone number is ____ ."

Doctors recommend that patients with chronic illnesses such as diabetes or epilepsy wear identification bracelets with the essential information on them. It is also a good idea to carry a card in your wallet that identifies your diagnosis, the name of your doctor, and whom to call in an emergency.

Once you're there, roll with the punches. You're going to witness tough situations—that's what the emergency room is for. The attitudes of the staff may not seem sensitive or humane, but those professionals are probably working under conditions where sensitivity may be a luxury and is not always feasible. Emergency room medicine, by definition, is task oriented. Doctors and nurses are required to work under constant pressure and may be so drained that they may not be able to express as much compassion as you might expect under other circumstances—remember that their job is to save lives and take care of acute crises. So if you're truly in doubt or if you feel what's bothering you is too urgent or frightening to wait until the next week, it's better to prepare yourself, be patient, and bring a friend or a good book. You are your own advocate and must take charge of your own health.

Some conditions do go away on their own, but others may get worse and even put you in jeopardy. If you really don't know what to do, call your doctor's office and describe your symptoms. If your doctor is unavailable, you are probably better off taking the cautious approach and making the visit, even if it's in the middle of the night.

Why Don't I Want to Go See My Doctor?

It's tough to admit to yourself that you are sick. When you've had a symptom for a while, you begin to agonize—should you or shouldn't you go? You really don't want to. We all feel inadequate anyway, and hate to face the doctor because our health habits are not as good as we know they should be. And when we go to the doctor, we have to face all that. That's why a few days before an appointment, some overweight patients go on fierce diets, those with hypertension may cut down on salt, and many people brush their teeth harder and longer than usual and floss three times a day.

Unfortunately, these days there are lots of anxieties and little gratification involved in visiting the doctor. In our youth-oriented culture, good health is considered almost a virtue, which is why everybody feels inadequate when they do get sick, especially if it happens frequently. You can't go into a bookstore, watch a commercial, or read an ordinary magazine without being confronted with pictures of splendid specimens burgeoning with good health. When I was a guest on a talk show, a man called in and began telling me everything that he hated about going to the doctor. I asked him when he did go to the doctor, and he replied,

> *"Only when I want to find out what's wrong with me. When I want to feel better, I go to my chiropractor."*

Before we had all the high-tech procedures, doctors mostly offered measures aimed at symptom relief such as herbal medicines, special teas, nutritious potions, poultices, and compresses. Rich patients went to spas for their annual "cure," took the mineral baths, and enjoyed the massages. Even if these "cures" were ineffective, they were all meant to help the patient feel better. Today when you go to the doctor, the tests you are subjected to and the prescriptions you are given are not likely to make you feel better for at least a day or two. And most doctors do not pay a lot of attention to the immediate relief of your symptoms.

One of the reasons people often procrastinate about making a doctor's appointment is that they fear having to undergo very unpleasant, sometimes painful, and usually expensive diagnostic procedures. Lab tests are almost invariably a major feature of visiting the doctor. You have to entrust your-self to a series of unknown assistants. Even producing a urine specimen is demeaning. You struggle to furnish just the right amount (and not more!) and the whole process makes you unusually self-conscious about one of your natural functions. Then comes the blood drawing. Despite reassurances to the contrary from the technician, it often hurts and you try not to flinch. And if it doesn't go smoothly, you may be the one who gets blamed:

"Oops, I'll have to try again. Has anyone else ever told you that your veins are hard to hit? You have such small veins!"

After that, having the inevitable X rays and EKG, although less un-comfortable, is still time consuming and may seem ominous. The so-called "stress test" is accurately named; it's frightening to find yourself exercising undressed on a treadmill with measuring devices attached to your body and egged on to persist as long as you possibly can hold out. Then there is another whole set of tests justifiably referred to as "invasive" and which may be "uncomfortable." Inform yourself so that you will be forewarned and forearmed.

So, When Do You Really Have To Go?

Certain conditions are clear-cut and present no problem in judgment to either patient or doctor. Trauma is clearly defined; everybody knows what's wrong and that something has to be done. If you break a leg or cut yourself badly, you will have no hesitation in going to see a doctor. But for illnesses and lesser injuries, the decision is less obvious and it is difficult to formu-late a good guideline. It's impossible to list all the eventualities that make visiting the doctor a desirable thing to do. There may be a symptom that, even if it occurs only once, is serious enough for you to go to the doctor. And certainly any noticeable changes in your bodily function such as persistent pain or a symptom you don't expect or understand is enough to merit seeing a doctor.

Deciding when to go is a balance between how sick you feel and your fear of going to the doctor. People have been misled into believing that a "real" illness comes with an elevation of temperature. But many serious illnesses require medical attention even though they are not accompanied by fever. Unfortunately, some patients are discouraged from visiting the doctor for fear of being ridiculed or appearing hypochondriacal. They postpone calling until it is too late and often end up in the emergency room, taken care of by professionals they have never seen before. You have to remember that consulting a doctor is not a disgrace or an admission of failure. It certainly isn't your fault that you are sick, even though some people seem to try to make you feel that way and even though you may, at times, feel that way yourself.

Although there are no hard and fast rules about when to consult a doctor, if you are not sure, it's best to call and find out. Just because you don't have a fever doesn't mean you shouldn't go to the doctor—that's foolish. Also, just because someone says, *"When I had that I was all right after a few days,"* or tells you it's not serious, or somebody else's doctor told them it wasn't necessary to come in when they had similar symptoms—those are not valid reasons. There are a great number of medical conditions that necessitate medical attention but have symptoms that are not that apparent. Between the serious, threatening conditions and minor illnesses, there is a wide range of malfunctions that benefit from medical attention. If you are worried about a symptom, no matter how seemingly minor, such as a cough or headache, call the doctor. The peace of mind is worth it, and it will help you in the future if the symptom returns.

All of us have unique expectations that influence our decisions about when to see the doctor. You may ask your physician what is serious enough to justify a telephone call between appointments, but even if your doctor is willing, it will be difficult for anyone to give you a fail-safe set of criteria. A certain amount of insight into your own attitudes and behavior about health and illness will be valuable to you.

A young woman who plays a lot of tennis and always walks up the stairs instead of taking elevators suddenly finds herself less able to do this; she becomes alarmed:

"I was perfectly able to do this before, there must be something wrong with my heart."

Another person who doesn't expect to be able to walk up four flights of stairs without panting would never consider this a reason to consult a physician. Similarly, if you have a perfect record of never missing a day's work, and find yourself not able to go one day, you may feel you have a serious problem. Another person might have a less rigid work ethic:

"I need a couple of mental health days because I've been under too much stress lately."

There are environmental factors and past experiences that sensitize patients. Someone with a family history of a particular disease may become alarmed by symptoms another person might not even notice. A patient who realizes that he is getting up more at night to go to the bathroom ends up thinking, *"I remember, that's what happened to Dad. I better go and have myself tested,"* because his father has diabetes. Or a parent who heard a story on the evening news about a child who had convulsions from high fever might then overreact when her own child develops chills and fever. In some cases, these situations can lead to misunderstandings with your doctor. Not knowing why you are reacting so strongly, you may be judged as an overanxious patient unless you make a point of explaining why you are so worried.

It is important to think of physicians as not only being there to treat us when we are sick, but also for preventing illness. With the current emphasis on wellness care, doctors are there to keep us from becoming ill and teach us how to stay healthy. When you go to your physician, besides giving attention to your immediate needs, your doctor should advise you on your diet, recommend a desirable amount of physical exercise, advise how to avoid some of the harmful environments such as passive smoke or sun exposure, and help you understand better how your body functions.

Making the Appointment

You agonize over making the decision and then finally call your doctor. At first you are relieved that you have done the right thing. Then you begin to have doubts again. It's very common for patients to tell us that they begin to feel better as soon as they've called the doctor. And some are embarrassed because when they arrive for the appointment, their symptoms seem to disappear. They question whether the decision to consult the doctor was wise or even necessary. Don't feel that way! If your symptom concerns you enough for you to call the doctor, then you need to be there.

Even picking up the phone to make the call is not as simple as it used to be. How often have you been subjected to a computerized voice listing endless push-button options? Nowadays, in self-defense, some people have learned to pretend that they don't have touch-tone phones in the hope of being able to speak with a real live human being. Answering services are so impersonal:

> *"The doctor is out for the weekend. If you leave a message on the voice mail, Dr. SoAndSo will return your call as soon as possible."*

Patients leave messages and don't know whether they should wait to see if a doctor will call back or whether they need to go to an emergency room. Sometimes patients are informed,

> *"The doctor is out of the office; we will beep him for you."*

Hours go by and no one calls back. Even when the doctor is in, what patients usually hear on the telephone is,

> *"Doctor is with a patient now,"*

and are then placed on hold. A frequent complaint:

> *"I'd been on hold for at least five minutes when I heard this click and then the dial tone. I'd been disconnected again!"*

Once you've gotten up your courage to call, it's disappointing to learn that you will not be seen for a while:

"We won't be able to fit you in until three weeks from now, on the twenty-third at 2:45."

What if you're really not feeling well? If you think it's important for your health to be seen promptly, you must insist on being seen earlier. But, if you cannot wait for the appointment, you should be prepared for the suggestion that you see the doctor's partner. Or you may be told that when you get there you will have to wait longer than usual. It may simply not be possible for them to schedule time with your own doctor when he or she is already heavily booked. What if the only appointment you are offered is on the day that you have an important meeting? Or if it's at the time you have to pick up your children at school? Do you ask for a different day and time, or must you just take what you can get? You have to ask yourself:

"Does the medical appointment have priority? What are the consequences if I delay? What are my options?"

The Waiting Room

You probably move heaven and earth to get to your appointments on time. You allow for traffic and parking because you don't want to be late. If you're lucky, when you get there, the receptionist knows you and greets you pleasantly, and the doctor is waiting to see you. Unfortunately, with the pressures that exist in the current health-care system, this is the exception and not the rule. An angry patient recently walked out of a doctor's office saying:

"In that office, it seems like time doesn't mean a thing if it's other people's time. It was a whole hour today. I wouldn't have minded if they told me it would be an hour. Why couldn't they tell me that?"

All too often, a harried receptionist abruptly hands you a clipboard with pages of standardized questions, and you navigate your way through a packed waiting room with a lonely, uncomfortable feeling of alienation. In this next, unfortunately quite typical scenario, the receptionist is behind the admitting desk talking to a patient on the phone:

> RECEPTIONIST: *Mr. Johnson, I have you down for the tenth. I explained that to you yesterday. It's the tenth not the eleventh.* (Phone rings) *Let me put you on hold, I have another call. Yes, this is Alicia. Yes I do have space on the nineteenth.* (Another line rings) *I'm sorry, my line again, let me put you on hold.*

Then someone knocks on the frosted window:

> RECEPTIONIST: *I'll get to you as soon as I can. Just have a seat.*
>
> PATIENT: *But, I—*

Before allowing the patient to finish her sentence, the receptionist shuts the partition. When she gets off the phone, she opens the window again.

> RECEPTIONIST: *I'm afraid there will be a longish wait before the doctor will see you.*
>
> PATIENT: *But I spoke with the doctor earlier today and he told me to come on in.*
>
> RECEPTIONIST: *You'll have to be more patient. That's right, we'll get you in as soon as possible, but it's still going to be a wait. There are other patients waiting who were here before you. So just be patient. I'll let the nurse know you're here.*

Patients are often discouraged before they even see the doctor. The forms you are asked to complete require information from your drivers' license number and your mother's maiden name to details about your health history, some of which you are unable to answer:

> *Have you ever had a reaction to . . . ?*
> *Have you ever experienced . . . ?*
> *Are you allergic to . . . ?*
> *Are there any members of your family who . . . ?*
> *When did you first notice . . . ?*

THE DOCTOR GETS A DOSE OF HER OWN MEDICINE

Recently, after I was hospitalized for treatment of an injured leg, I was given an appointment for follow-up in the office of my orthopedist. I suffered through two hours of one unnecessary inconvenience and putdown after another. I was so indignant about the way I was treated that I told my doctor I would never visit his office again. He asked me to write him a letter summarizing my experience, and so I did. I was aware of how busy he was, so I wrote it in an almost shorthand style:

> Dear Dr. _____:
>
> I told you I would never return to your office . . . if I could possibly avoid it. This has nothing to do with the excellent medical care I received from you personally for which I am most appreciative.

Notice that I paid him a compliment right up front. In writing a letter of complaint, it's not a good idea to be totally negative. You need to emphasize the positive aspects as well. Then, I introduced the problem:

> However, my recent office visit was a nightmare. I arrived for my eagerly awaited 2:45 visit exactly on time. My wheelchair was pushed into the waiting area with its high counter behind which several staff members were busy with one another or the phone. No one said hello and no one, at any time during my sojourn in the waiting area, ever looked at me or used my name.
>
> I spied a clipboard and dutifully signed in.
>
> Settled in the waiting area and seriously doubted whether anyone knew I was there. Tried to figure out strategy for reminding someone of my presence without annoying them.
>
> Realized that as a new patient in the office I would undoubtedly be required to fill out some insurance forms and repeat all the medical, historical data. Sent companion to counter, she managed to engage one of the staff long enough to acquire a second clipboard with all the necessary forms.
>
> Did my homework, but realized that someone in the hospital had failed to return my Medicare card. I did have the card for my supplemental insurance.

Initially, I didn't expect this would be a big problem. I knew that the doctor had the Medicare information from caring for me in the hospital the previous week. So I assumed that the necessary information could easily be gotten by looking at my hospital record. But that was not the case:

> Your assistant abruptly indicated that it was not her responsibility to get that information. When my friend attempted to appeal to her by stating that I was a physician, your assistant also loudly informed anyone within earshot, "Well, if she is a doctor, the least she could do is to know what she has to have in her purse when she comes to the office!"
>
> Asked at desk for an estimate of how much longer we would have to wait. The answer: "You won't know until the door opens and they call your name. There are several doctors here, you know."
>
> Finally, our big moment, and the door opens for us! A pleasant nurse greets me, knows who I am, that I am there, and why. Moreover, she explains that you had been taking care of two emergencies and a hospital admission for surgery.

That explanation satisfied me. But it should have come earlier.

> The problems I am describing could be so easily fixed. Someone needs to say hello, look at you, maybe even indicate that they are there to help you. If the wait is long, someone needs to acknowledge that you are there, that you are waiting, that they are sorry, and give you some idea of what's going on behind that wall and that door that so rigidly separate the "we" and "they" of the medical establishment.
>
> None of these interventions takes time, they don't cost money, they simply require an awareness of the patient as a person. We have paid lip service to this concept for so long a time that it has become a platitude! But we are not heeding it. On the short haul, the disempowering experiences I describe will be accepted by patients who are dependent on the physician for care, but not for long, especially in the present medical climate.

In writing this letter, as a doctor, I was able to take certain liberties. But, you also have options when you encounter injustices and inefficiencies. Anyone can complain. Anyone can make suggestions. Find out who will be the most responsive to your concerns. But don't be on the attack for things you don't understand. First try to understand them. The doctor is accountable to you. Changes can be made. In fact, when I relented and did return to this doctor's office, the treatment I received from the staff was definitely improved.

I was careful not to say anything bad about any individual person in that office. I never said,

"Your receptionist was rude or SoAndSo didn't look at me."

If you have complaints, stick to the experience and not the person who caused it:

"Why is it that when you've already given all that information at the hospital registration desk, you have to give it all again here?"

Instead of,

"That woman in the brown jacket at the reception desk was really rude and told me that I had to . . ."

Find out about the procedure. If you have a personal complaint about someone in particular, then you need to handle it very gingerly. Try to keep complaints impersonal and make constructive suggestions about the experience itself.

Most patients acquiesce when given instructions at the front window, but it's important to know that if you do feel in need of urgent help, you must speak up. The receptionist may be so busy with calls that she unintentionally ignores you, and the doctors are almost always busy with patients and unaware of what's going on in the waiting room.

When I complained about what happened, my physician said, *"Please tell me what's wrong so I can fix it!"* He actually encouraged me to write because he wanted documentation of what his office was like for patients so that he could educate his staff.

In some cases you may not want to burden the doctor, but it would always be legitimate to ask for the name of the person you should speak to or address a letter of complaint. Depending on your doctor's style of running the practice, he or she may either want to know the details or not. Not all doctors are likely to welcome being told how to run their offices.

Remember that at this time in health care, physicians' offices are marketing their services and your responses are extremely important. Make yourself heard if you feel you have a legitimate concern. Ask the doctor whom to talk to. There may be times when things seem unnecessarily cumbersome—but before you attack, try to find someone to explain why.

Giving Your Medical History

This is often the most important part of the medical visit for you and your doctor. It is necessary in helping the doctor make a correct diagnosis. Depending on how well your doctor knows you, there may be a few questions concerning your recent health and well-being, or it may be necessary to take a complete history starting from the beginning. You may find yourself annoyed by all the questions that allow only "yes" or "no" answers. Being curt may be useful to the doctor for certain parts of the medical history. Still, all the problems in the doctor–patient relationship and communication, which are the subject of so much interest, research, and teaching, do influence how effective the medical history taking will be. On both sides of the equation, good communication skills will result in a better medical history.

I've heard so many patients complain about having to give the same answers over and over. They have filled out forms. They may have already told the same things to the doctor who referred them to the new doctor they are seeing now, and then they have to explain it all over again to the receptionist, to the nurse, and finally once more to the doctor. Having to repeat information can rob it of its reality or importance. If you're at a party and someone doesn't hear what you have just said and asks you,

"What did you say?"

You may find yourself replying,

"Never mind—it wasn't important."

Having made the statement one time makes you wonder whether it was worth saying again even though the other person may desperately want to know what you said. It even makes you question the validity of what you're saying. This is also true in the doctor's office. When you've already explained your symptoms to the receptionist, then the nurse, and finally when the doctor comes in and says, *What are you here for today?* you begin to wonder:

Is what I'm saying really worthwhile?

But don't let that stop you. It's important for your doctor to hear the story of your illness directly from you in your own words, and to listen to you express your concerns and give all the relevant information. Your description may alert the doctor to crucial issues that would otherwise have gone unnoticed. This is also a good time to voice some of your more personal concerns. Realize that your doctor deals with many different people who all have different ways of behaving. Some patients are so defensive and tough that they don't let on how badly they really feel. Others react very dramatically to illness and tend to overstate their complaints. Let the doctor know the type of patient you are:

"I may come across to you as pretty nervous about this lump, but so many people in my family have had breast cancer . . . ."

If you know yourself to be stoical, the doctor needs to know that too:

"I'm not the type to complain. I really have a high pain threshold."

Have you ever felt the need to debunk your symptoms?

"This is probably nothing serious but it never happened to me before."
"I have been so tired. I know lots of people are tired but I've just never felt this way before."
"You'll probably tell me it's nothing to worry about."

These long statements serve no function; in fact, they are really only apologies for being sick.

A common source of misunderstanding is when patients block the appropriate empathetic response from the doctor by prematurely explaining their symptoms instead of describing them. It's difficult for all of us to acknowledge a symptom without simultaneously attributing a cause to it. Even for ordinary colds, people try to figure out why:

> *"Whom did I catch this from?"*
> *"Where did I go that I might have picked this up?"*
> *"What did I do that might have brought this on?"*

And with limited medical knowledge, patients may come up with explanations that often make no sense whatsoever. Then they feel bad when the doctor rejects their explanation. In the novel *Buddenbrooks*, Nobel prize-winning author Thomas Mann describes a young man who drives his friends and acquaintances crazy because he keeps complaining that he is in constant pain. He is sure that all the nerves on the left side of his body are too short. He goes on and on about how these short nerves must be what cause him his persistent, vague, indescribable but agonizing torment.

Sometimes what you come up with just doesn't make sense to a doctor. And when this happens, doctors become terribly frustrated. If, for instance, every time you have a minor symptom, you rush to the doctor suspecting a major calamity,

> *"Oh doctor, I think I must be getting a heart attack. Every time I eat I get this feeling in my chest,"*

even a well-meaning, sympathetic doctor is going to debunk what you have to say, instead of giving the response you had hoped:

> *"My goodness, whatever made you think that you're having a heart attack every time you feel uncomfortable after a large meal?"*

Offering fanciful theories to explain your symptoms can really put your doctor on the spot. The patient who self-diagnoses and then initiates his or her own treatment, which does not make medical sense, can trigger negative responses from the doctor. The doctor has two choices—humor the patient and go along with what he or she is saying, or argue with the patient, which is hard because the doctor argues on the basis of medical science while the patient counters with personal experiences. Giving an honest explanation carries the risk of making patients feel put down and suggests that the doctor was not sympathetic.

In some instances your theory and what you are doing about your symptoms, although inappropriate, are intrinsically harmless and the doctor may not challenge you. If, for instance, you say,

"Since I started taking vitamin C, I feel like a new person."

The doctor may not argue with you, even though taking vitamin C will have no immediate effect on the way you feel each day. Another patient who had noticed a loose tooth claimed:

"I decided to try taking calcium tablets and after only two or three days, my tooth wasn't loose anymore."

Here again, a few days of calcium will not reattach a loose tooth to the underlying bone, but the doctor went along with it. How would you feel if you found out that your doctor had essentially humored you instead of arguing with you?

In yet one more typical encounter, a patient had formulated her own theories as to why she felt shaky after eating candy:

"I get a sugar rush after I eat sweets and then I get low blood sugar and I have to eat right away."

A common belief patients have is that if they eat something very sweet and rich, say a large chocolate bar, that a few hours later their blood sugar will be abnormally low. Most patients with such complaints have been tested and have not been found to have abnormally low blood sugar unless they are inherently diabetic. In this case, the doctor felt that he had to challenge his patient's theory because he had already tested her blood sugar level, found it to be normal, and he was concerned that her beliefs could lead to undesirable eating habits:

DOCTOR: *No, I'm afraid that's not true. You do not have hypoglycemia—*

PATIENT: *But I always feel so shaky after eating something sweet, I can feel that my blood sugar level is very low . . . .*

DOCTOR: *But it's not because your blood sugar is low. When you feel like that, it means . . . .*

This doctor tried to convince the patient that she was wrong. He was caught in a bind between arguing against or accepting what this patient had to say. If you are in a situation where you really want to know whether the doctor agrees with you or not, then ask:

"Some people tell me my blood sugar is low. Do you think that's true? Why do I feel that way after I eat sweets?"

Or,

"It seems like since I've been taking vitamin C, I feel better. Does that make sense to you? Could that be the case?"

Although you can't expect your doctor to accept an explanation that does not make medical sense, you still hope for a sympathetic response to your suffering. Don't argue. Show that you are trying to understand. Give your doctor the opportunity to explain things by asking:

"What does it mean when I feel like that? I've heard that when people get this kind of pain, it means they have . . . . <u>Is that true</u>?"

The Physical Examination

Physical examinations make everyone anxious. In our society, touching the body of another person is sanctioned only under very special circumstances. And the physical examination breaks a lot of the taboos about strangers touching one another. In addition, almost every part of the examination suggests to the patient that the doctor may find something wrong. If a doctor carefully palpates your breasts, going through your mind is,

Do I have breast cancer?

Or if the doctor listens to your chest for longer than usual, you ask yourself,

Why is he doing that? Is there something he is worrying about?

During any part of the exam, you figure the doctor wouldn't be looking carefully unless there might be something wrong. So besides being embarrassing and uncomfortable, the exam is also frightening.

Traditionally, the physical examination was the time of closest direct contact between patient and physician. But more and more, physicians are resorting to instrumentation and high-tech methods for the examination. Although the stethoscope was invented by Laënnec early in the nineteenth century, physicians practiced "direct auscultation" for the first few decades of this century. This meant that they placed their ear directly on the patient's chest to hear the heartbeat and the sounds of the lungs. Now, complex technology is used to examine the heart and the lungs, which far exceeds the tapping and listening that some of us remember. It has been said that the stethoscope is almost an obsolete instrument, even though it has become the stereotype for the medical professional. While all the technical advances lead to much more precise diagnoses—X rays and CT scans are more accurate than the traditional examination—these tests increase the social distance between doctor and patient, making patients feel as if they are being kept at arm's length.

Another way that the physical examination has been depersonalized is that it is now universally required for physicians and other health professionals to wear rubber gloves. The reason for the widespread use of gloves is to protect patient and physician from exposure to some prevalent infections that can be easily transmitted. But gloves may constitute a barrier to the healing touch. There is something about seeing your physician carefully putting gloves on before getting near you that makes you feel,

What are they afraid of catching from me? What might they be afraid of giving me?

One hospitalized patient commented:

"The nurse's aides who came in to give me a basin for my morning bed bath would hand that basin to me only after putting gloves on with care. Some of them would only take my blood pressure if they had gloves on. It made me feel like Typhoid Mary!"

For patients with chronic illness, especially those who have conditions such as HIV, the use of rubber gloves causes them to feel progressively alienated. One dying patient poignantly described her feelings:

> "I am alone. I am alone and I am lonely. I hold one of my hands in the other, to feel some warmth. But my hands are cold. I grasp my left wrist with my right hand. I rub the fingers of my left hand over my right arm. I must touch myself to feel any warmth because no one else will touch me without the gloves. Everyone is afraid of me . . . . I have one desire. I have one hope. I hope that someone, anyone, will remove one glove and hold my hand before I die. I hope that someone will come in and sit by my side and take off one glove and touch my hand. I hope that someone will take off one glove—just for a moment—and touch me."[2]

A large part of the physical, as well as other procedures, is often carried out without any explanation or running commentary about what is happening. This can also make it more painful than it needs to be. Certain procedures necessitate the doctor or technician's concentration and they are not able to pay much attention to the patient's responses. In reviewing videotaped medical encounters, we have noticed that patients often raise important issues while the doctor is listening to their chest with the stethoscope. Why? It is one of the only times during the examination when the doctor is completely silent and the patient has a chance to talk.

A friend told of his wife's recent visit to an acupuncturist. She was satisfied and mentioned among other things that the practitioner explained everything he did while he was doing it. In response, the husband stated wistfully:

> "I wish my doctors and dentists would do that. They never tell me what they are doing or how long it is going to take, and I'd sure feel better if they did. Even if they only said, 'We're about halfway through now.'"

Why didn't he ask them to do that? He told me that it had never occurred to him. I asked if he thought his doctor would mind. "No," he said, "she would probably like it if I told her my preferences." Yet he had never thought of that option. Later, I told the anecdote to another friend, who is more aggressive and outspoken than most. She thought for a moment and then surprised me by stating that even she would probably also not venture to speak up. So much for patient autonomy.

How do you feel when your physician does not explain anything during the physical? As patients, we all must remember to speak up for ourselves. If you must undergo a procedure, ask the doctor beforehand whether he or she would be able to give you an idea of what needs to be done and how long it may take. Then, during the procedure, ask about how it is progressing. Remember that, as the doctor is doing the physical examination, especially while listening to your chest, it may not be possible to be attentive to what you are saying. So if you suddenly remember something you forgot when you gave your medical history, bide your time and relay the information at a time when your doctor can note it.

During the physical, doctors may ask questions they have never asked before or pay extra attention to a certain part of the examination. One patient, Susan, came home after a visit to the doctor and her husband Jim inquired about how it had gone.

> *"It went fine, he gave me a real thorough exam,"* Susan began, *"except . . . ."*
>
> *"Except what?"* Jim asked.
>
> *"Well, it just seemed like he listened to my chest for a long time. I was really scared whether anything was wrong."*
>
> *"Well, didn't you ask?"*
>
> *"Oh, no,"* Susan said, *"I didn't think it was my business to ask questions about the way he examined me and he didn't say anything. I would have felt stupid asking."*

When you are asked further specific questions during part of the physical examination, it's natural to think that it has some ominous relationship to what the doctor is observing. If, for instance, a doctor is examining a young woman's abdomen and he stops to ask her about her menstrual cycle, she may begin to wonder whether he has found a cyst or some more serious problem. But it may simply be that he forgot to ask when he was taking the medical history. That's the time when you, as the patient, should inquire why he's asking so that you don't go home and lose sleep.

There may be times during the physical examination when more information and an honest explanation could save patients unnecessary anxiety. One patient, Betty, recently remarked,

> *"I went to my internist for a regular checkup and after the technician took my blood pressure, he stopped and repeated taking my blood pressure. Then he asked me if I was taking blood pressure medication. It frightened me. His question seemed like a suggestion that I should be on medication."*

For the rest of the visit, until Betty was able to talk to her doctor, she experienced unnecessary anxiety and her blood pressure was probably rising higher. Had she had the courage to interrupt and ask, *"Well, what is my blood pressure?"* she might have felt better. Because later when she did ask, she was told that it was borderline and that all she had to do was get a little more exercise.

There are reasons why patients don't ask their doctors when they are concerned. Sometimes it's because they are afraid and don't want to know. But if there is something you don't understand during the physical examination, then by all means ask about it:

> *"Why are you listening for so long? Is there something that doesn't sound good about my heart?"*

If you don't want to interrupt, be sure to ask about any aspect that was alarming before you leave:

> *"You seemed to be palpating my abdomen with more care than usual— is there something that I should know about?"*

Usually, patients aren't told what their blood pressure is or given other details of the examination unless they ask. Sometimes nurses and physicians hesitate because it involves a lot of explanation and they worry that the patient may take it too seriously. There is, in fact, nothing about the findings the doctor or nurse obtains during the examination that you don't have a right to know. It is usually preferable to wait until the end of the examination, unless it just works out better for you to talk about your concern immediately.

Your doctor should encourage you to get better informed, but it's up to you to make the attempt. Ask the question, and don't try to guess. Forget about apologizing. Your fears are fueling your imagination, and you have the right to know the results of your physical. Ideally, after the examination you should have the opportunity to sit down with the doctor in the consultation room fully dressed and discuss your questions. Make sure that your expectations from the visit have been met and that you understand what you are told.

▾ Did your doctor explain your symptoms or illness to you?

▾ Do you understand the purpose of the medications you have been given?

▾ When and how are you to take them?

▾ Are there any possible side effects?

▾ If you had special concerns when you arrived, have they been responded to?

▾ Do you know what to expect between now and your next appointment?

▾ Did you learn something about yourself and your health?

WHEN YOUR CHILD
IS SICK

▼▼
▼▼

"What is he going to do to me?"
"How long is it going to take?"
"Let's not go today, I feel better. Let's wait until tomorrow."

Sound familiar? Many adults have similar thoughts, but they're too embarrassed to express them. When you decide to take your child to the pediatrician, you must consider some special issues. The child patient needs to be the focus of the planning as well as the visit. It is hardly ever the child's idea to go to the doctor and children are outspoken and honest in letting you know that. Listen carefully to your child. Sometimes you will hear fears and misconceptions about the medical visit that you may be able to dispel. If your child says,

"My friend Danny said when he went to the doctor, he took all his blood out,"

take this opportunity to explain that they will just take a tiny drop to make sure he's healthy.

How long ahead of time should you mention the appointment? That all depends on your child's level of comprehension. For the youngest children, up to four years of age, it is best not to start them worrying too early. If you begin preparing them on Monday and then try to reassure them by saying, *"Well, we're not going until Thursday,"* they may not even have a very clear idea when Thursday is going to come and may work themselves into a frazzle of anxiety. But even if you don't do it until the morning of the scheduled visit, you need to prepare and warn your child. All of us do better if we can prepare ourselves before going to the doctor, especially young children who are even less resilient because they have not yet developed their coping skills.

What Do You Tell Your Child?

Tell the truth. In the beginning, focus on familiar things that are easy to understand. The ride in the car, the elevator, the waiting room, the toys or books that will be waiting at the doctor's office to play with, the facts of having to be undressed, and what the doctor and the nurse will do. But nothing elaborate is really needed to prepare for the ordinary office visit. A picture book about going to the doctor can help. A toy doctor set often helps your child master the experience. Your presence and your honesty are what will help the most. Explain why people go to the doctor for checkups. Children tend to think unpleasant things are done to punish them because they have been bad. They need to know that everyone goes to the doctor, and that it is not because they have done something wrong. It also sometimes helps to tell the child the doctor's name so that it will be more familiar by the time you get there. Dr. Greentree sounds less formidable than *The Doctor.* Also stress to your child that you both will be returning to home base soon: *"After we finish, we'll go home for lunch."*

"Am I going to have any shots? Is it going to hurt?"

These are tough questions. Above all, although it may seem to make things easier at the time, make no promises that you cannot keep. It is essential that your child trust you not to lie, especially in a crisis. If you don't know what is going to happen, be honest and say so. But if you do, explain it in as nonthreatening a way as possible in a language that is familiar to children. You know what your child will understand. If, for instance, your child does not understand what a stethoscope is for, you might say something like,

"The doctor has something that's like a little telephone to listen to your chest."

It's a good idea to explain the different parts of the examination:

"The doctor has a special light to look inside your ear. He will probably ask you to open your mouth very wide, stick you tongue out, and pant like a dog. If you do that well, he will be able to see the back of your throat. If you don't, he might have to use a little flat stick to help him look."

> *The doctor will poke around your stomach a little. It may tickle a little. He will also take a little soft hammer and tap your knee with it—it won't hurt, but it will make your leg kick."*

It is especially difficult to prepare children honestly, but not too menacingly for the required injections. There's a good deal of controversy over the word "shot." Unfortunately, it is the word most children are used to. Sometimes it is better to use less frightening words:

"Yes, the doctor will probably have to give you a little stick today to keep you from getting sick. You may feel a pinch or something like a mosquito bite."

How do you prepare your child if it's an unexpected visit? Suppose your child develops a fever in the night and you are told to come in first thing in the morning. The same general principles apply. Tell him or her what you know in a language that is easy to comprehend as soon as you are able to:

"We are going to the doctor to find out why you feel bad and help you get better."

Ask the doctor or nurse on the phone what you might do ahead of time to make your son or daughter comfortable without interfering with the diagnosis. Although medication might bring a fever down or lessen abdominal pain, it may make it harder for the doctor to assess just how sick your child really is.

The Doctor's Office

What do you do when you're in the waiting room and everyone else's children are playing quietly while yours throws himself on the floor kicking and screaming?

"I won't go in there, I won't go in there! You can't make me!"

It seems as if everyone is suddenly looking at you, shocked at your inability to control your own child. You are mortified and desperate and will do almost anything to stop the behavior. Parents are sometimes tempted to threaten:

"If you don't stop, I will tell the doctor and he will _____ ."

Or,

"If you are bad, I will tell the doctor to give you a shot!"

Or, worse yet,

"If you keep acting like that, I'm going to tell the doctor to keep you here!"

Never use the doctor as a threat. Even if you're feeling exasperated and helpless in the face of an uncontrollable temper tantrum, it is better to let yourself be embarrassed than to use threats. Threats are a negative and dishonest way of preparing a child for what the doctor has to do; they create the impression that the child is at the doctor's because he or she is bad and is being punished. Don't waste your energy adding to your anxiety by wondering,

If I can't control my own child, how will the doctor be able to?

Even though you think it's going to be a knock-down, drag-out fight, very often you will be pleasantly surprised. There is something calming about the doctor's aura of authority and the fact that the doctor is not emotionally involved and probably very used to children who act up. If you start out feeling that you have been a failure before you even go in to see the doctor, it is not going to facilitate communication.

For many years, I had a wonderful tomcat named Blackie who was very wild and always in trouble. When he got hurt, if we were able to capture him, we would take him to a nearby veterinarian. One time he came home with a terrible injury to his eye. My husband and I finally caught him and, because he was raging mad, we put him in a cage in the trunk of my car. The drive was short, but I heard all sorts of horrible banging noises coming from the trunk and realized that he had opened the cage and was loose. When I got to the vet's, I didn't dare open the trunk because I was afraid Blackie would get out and take off down the road. So I went into the waiting room without him and found myself surrounded by well-behaved kittycats, dogs sitting quietly beside their masters, and all the smug and content animal owners. Suddenly, the receptionist called my name loudly across the waiting room and, when she spotted me, asked incredulously,

"Where's your pet?" Heads turned. Everyone's eyes were on me.

"Well, he's in the car," I replied sheepishly. The receptionist paused.

"Well, why didn't you bring him in?" she asked.

"I couldn't," was all I could say.

"What do you mean, you can't?" she asked. I told her that I was afraid to take him out of the trunk. I really felt foolish, and embarrassed. All these other sleek pets and their "parents" who could control them looked on, and there I was. The vet's assistant came out wearing big leather gloves and holding a net. She skillfully put the netting over the trunk and opened it. This was obviously not the first time she had had this experience. She reached in, grabbed hold of Blackie, and once in her arms, he lay down quietly like a baby.

"And you thought you wouldn't be able to handle this perfectly well-behaved cat!" she joked. Although the assistant treated my situation with humor, I felt like a total failure as an animal parent! All my self-confidence had dissolved and I even believed that the veterinarian's response to me would be jaded before we started.

While some parents are embarrassed when their child misbehaves in the waiting room, on the opposite end of spectrum are parents who bring in a child who constantly does things at home that are worrisome and then acts like an angel at the pediatrician's office. Perhaps your daughter won't sit still and listen at home or maybe your son has been having temper tantrums at the supermarket. But the doctor sees none of this and comments,

"As I have observed him here, he has been nice and quiet."

You then find yourself in the position of having to convince the doctor that there is a problem. Have you ever gone to the dentist because of a throbbing tooth that suddenly stops hurting the moment you reach the office? What can you do? Before the visit, decide what behaviors you would like to discuss with the doctor and the particular scenarios that best illustrate the problem. For instance, does the behavior usually happen during dinner, on the way to school, at bedtime, when other children are visiting, in a public place? Ideally, parents usually pray for their children to behave well at the doctor's office, so be thankful if this does happen. Then, when you speak with the doctor after the examination, express your concerns:

"I know Tom was well behaved here today, but when we are at home, he gets very angry when . . . He does this three or four times a day. . . . Is this normal?"

More often, children are anxious when they go to the doctor and tend to act up. Parents also tend to be anxious, which is sensed by the child. Small children, by their very nature, tend to get into everything and may disrupt office routine. If your child behaves badly in the office, do not be embarrassed or feel you have to assure the doctor,

"This never happens at home!"

Instead, use the occasion for problem solving. It may be an occasion for you to get some help with your child's behavior:

"Doctor, is it normal for him to do this at this age? How shall I best handle it?"

What Can You Do to Make the Visit Less Upsetting?

There are very few general rules except the need for sensitivity and kindness. In most instances, you will know what is best to do. For a scheduled appointment, organize your thoughts ahead of time and prioritize your questions and concerns. When you actually get to the office, you may be so preoccupied with reassuring your child and with other immediate happenings that you are unable to concentrate on your own agenda. Remember that you are there to be helped, not to impress the doctor with what a perfect parent you are.

You know your child's history, how shy or adventurous he or she is, what causes tears, what can bring a laugh, what expressions he or she uses to describe various body parts or bodily functions. So although you should allow your child to form a direct relationship with the doctor, you should also translate and mediate when needed. If, for instance, you know that your daughter's anxiety will mount while you talk to the doctor, ask if she may be allowed to play in the waiting room until it is time for the actual examination. When it comes to the examination, if there is something in particular that you think will be upsetting to your child, ask the doctor whether it would be possible to leave it until last.

When in the examination room, it's important for both pediatrician and parent to be aware that at all times the child may be listening. Pediatricians inadvertently say things that children misunderstand. And parents say hurtful things in front of their children without realizing it:

> *"He has always been a bad sleeper. I haven't had a night's sleep since he was born. His brother, now, he always did everything at the right time."*

When possible, it is best to discuss touchy subjects when your child cannot hear them. But also be aware that sending your child out of the examination room is not always the best solution; not being able to stay in may cause your child to wonder,

> *What are they saying about me?*

Not only do children become curious, but they also think that bad things are going to be said about them if they are sent out of the room. If this is your only option, give a lot of reassurance:

> *"Debbie, you were very good! Now I need a moment to talk with the doctor and then we'll go home."*

The best place for a discussion is in the consultation room after the examination. If you came to the visit with your child alone, ask one of the office staff members for help so that you will have a few minutes of one-to-one with the doctor.

Make the Best Use of Your Time with the Doctor

It would be a good idea to find out early on in the visit how much time the doctor has set aside for you. One of the inequities of many medical visits is that the doctor knows how much time he or she has to spend while you have no idea. Ideally, the doctor should elicit your agenda for the visit and then let you know what the game plan is so that the time can be spent to mutual satisfaction. If your doctor just automatically goes into the routine for an eighteen-month checkup and does not explore your agenda, you can change that. If there is something you would like to discuss, don't procrastinate:

> *"Today, I especially would like you to watch her walk. She seems to be favoring her right leg."*

Even if the pediatrician seems very thorough, the mother is generally the closest and most accurate observer of the child and can help focus the examination.

Of course, it is not only the child who is anxious about the visit to the doctor—mothers are also anxious and often distracted. The following scenario is one that doctors observe all the time:

> *"Oh, doctor, there is just one more thing I have to ask you about."*

The mother says this just as the pediatrician is on his way out the door. He stops in his tracks and turns.

"What was that?"
    "Lately he has been wetting the bed almost every night. He never did that before."

The fact that this particular question was raised so late was not an accident. The mother was embarrassed and had to gather enough courage to ask. But now, the doctor, who may have been the soul of patience throughout the visit, has reached the end of his tether. His schedule is tight that day and he thinks he has finished the visit. Then, just as he is on his way out the door, he is asked a question to which there is no simple, short answer. That "one more thing" is often the straw that breaks the doctor's back.

Worse yet than the *"Oh, doctor, there's just one more thing"* is the tendency not to mention serious concerns at all because the parent is embarrassed or the doctor seems too busy to be bothered. We asked a series of parents as they were leaving the pediatrician's office what had been their main concerns before coming in and if they still had questions they had not asked. In response, over half the parents mentioned significant behavioral problems such as sleep disturbances, bed wetting, and thumb sucking that were really worrying them but which they had not mentioned. What were their reasons?

"The doctor doesn't want to be bothered with that."
"He's so busy."
"I'll ask someone else, maybe the teacher at the nursery."

There are various reasons why you may not bring up important things with the doctor—you might forget, you may be embarrassed, or perhaps you don't want to hear what the doctor will say. It is wise not to prejudge which problems the pediatrician can help you with. The questions you ask will help the doctor to understand your child and you better.

It's up to you to make sure that you understand what you are told and to ask questions when you do not. Don't be afraid to seem ignorant. It is too often assumed that just by being a parent you should know all about children. And everyone else acts like an expert—family, friends, and neighbors all tell you what to do:

"What I did with my child was I never let him . . . ."
"My sister let her daughter cry it out."
"Don't you think it would be better if you . . . ."

But these self-appointed consultants, although well intentioned, can only tell you about what worked for their own children; it may not work for yours. Keep in mind that each child is different and that no one knows your child as well as you do.

If you share the care of your child with a nanny or day-care staff member, let your doctor know the extent other caretakers are participating. A doctor needs to know the source of the information. One physician told me,

"I asked the mother a lot of detailed questions about the way she was feeding the baby and I only found out later that it was the grand-mother who usually handled the feeding."

Remember to get relevant information from the others involved in your child's care because they may have important observations. And after you see the doctor, be sure to let them know what the doctor's recommendations were because it may be up to them to carry them out.

It is your perfect right and—in fact, your responsibility—to ask for a second opinion whenever you are in doubt. Any pediatrician should be open to the idea that a parent will feel more comfortable in discussing an important decision with more than one expert. It not only reassures the parents but also the pediatrician who carries the burden of having to make many solitary decisions. However, any time you want a second opinion, it is advisable—in fact, almost mandatory—that you discuss it with your regular pediatrician before you seek out someone else. One of the things that really annoys physicians are parents who "doctor-shop." After consulting one pediatrician about a particular problem, some parents will then go to another and withhold what the original doctor said. Sometimes they do this just to check whether the new doctor will come up with the same answers. One young doctor who had just seen such a patient said:

> *"Sometimes you get a sense that parents are deliberately not forthcoming with information because they want to see if you [the doctor] will find out . . . that makes me mad because they're trying to trick me."*

Although there may be perfectly good reasons to consult more than one doctor about a problem, withholding information is a dishonest way of starting the relationship and, in the end, you will not get the best treatment. It's important to communicate openly and honestly about your child.

Am I an Overconcerned Parent?

Most physicians dread overconcerned parents because they make many demands and are difficult to satisfy. There is no parent who doesn't feel at times that the doctor thinks they are taking their child's complaints too seriously. And so it is natural to wonder whether you really are overconcerned. Physicians do expect the parents of newborns and very young babies to be anxious. But when children get a little older, the physician's attitude may change. While adults who go to the doctor every time they sneeze may be judged as hypochondriacs, the situation is more complicated in pediatrics. The whole dynamic of the relationship changes—it's hypochrondria once removed. Every time there is the slightest change, some parents panic and rush to the doctor. If you call frequently, then your pediatrician will have to screen your questions and complaints—some will be issues that actually require medical attention, others will be due to parental anxiety. Just as physicians who take care of adult patients tend to react negatively to those they perceive to be hypochondriacs, children's doctors may become less receptive to parents who are overconcerned. They will become impatient and sometimes even resentful of unexpected phone calls or requests for "urgent" appointments.

Parental overconcern can end up rubbing off on children and influence their health behavior. A study was conducted in a school in which the children, if they didn't feel well, were allowed to go directly to the school nurse without having to ask their teachers' permission.[1] It was discovered that those who went to the nurse most frequently were the children of parents who, although essentially well, were known to visit and call their doctors frequently. This group of patients are often referred to as the "worried well" and, in this study, their children had followed suit.

All pediatricians experience parents with "vulnerable" children who are not truly sick or at risk, but whose parents believe them to be. There are various reasons for behaving like an overconcerned parent. Some of these are "iatrogenic"—that is, they are caused by the physician's own behavior. Some physicians have a tendency to overreact to parents' complaints and, more important, are too ready to prescribe medication, other treatment, or do tests for symptoms that essentially are trivial. Too many children who have weekday bellyaches because they don't want to go to school end up having extensive examinations and tests. A parent who visits the pediatrician and finds that each complaint is met with some sort of diagnostic test or medical intervention—a prescription or other kind of treatment—may begin to take even the most minor problems more seriously than warranted. Studies have shown that early hospitalization, frequent changes of formula, and administration of medication for "normal" colic in infants all contribute to this phenomenon.

Other reasons for parents' perceiving their children as vulnerable can be found in their past experiences. If a family has lost a previous child, if the mother has had a miscarriage, if one of the family members, especially a child, has suffered from a serious illness, naturally the parents' responses to subsequent health problems will be exaggerated or at least changed.

So there may be perfectly valid reasons for you to be overconcerned. How many times are you allowed to call a pediatrician before you get labeled or are stigmatized as overanxious? There really is no clear definition, and so it is important to help the physician understand when you do feel especially anxious. Although a doctor may believe that a parent's repeated complaints are insignificant, the parent obviously has the opposite opinion. There is a fine line between having a physician who overreacts and one who debunks your complaints. Be sensitive to whether you think you are getting the appropriate response from the pediatrician. If your calls are not being returned and you are feeling rejected, ask your pediatrician whether he or she thinks you are overanxious. Enlist the physician's help in knowing when you really should be concerned.

How Can You Help During Painful Procedures?

What do you say if your child screams during an examination or an injection? Is it a good idea to tell your child not to cry? Many parents are tempted to do this out of fear of making a bad impression in the doctor's office. However, loud protests may actually be healthy and modern pediatricians are aware of this. So, don't say,

"Stop being a crybaby!"

And never promise that something is not going to hurt if it may actually be painful:

"Don't worry, you won't feel anything."

That will only cause your child to lose trust in you when he or she finds out that it actually does hurt. On the other hand, too much warning may act as a self-fulfilling prophesy:

"This is going to hurt"

may make things worse. You walk a thin line between frightening the child unduly and undermining trust with false reassurance. The truth is always best, choosing the least frightening words:

"This may bother you, you may feel it a little . . . ."

It helps to provide a distraction—anything that actively involves the child and keeps him or her from overreacting to the discomfort. Suggest counting and count along with your child. Tell him or her to take deep breaths, or even ask about a familiar bedtime story. Remember that these things are helpful for some children, but not necessarily for yours. You know your child best.

"Can I be with my child during the procedure?"

These days, it is usually permissible for the parent to be present in the room during procedures, preferably holding the child or just holding hands. In the past, it was believed that sending the mother out during procedures would make the child more cooperative. Parents used to be told dogmatically,

"He'll cry less if you're not in the room."

However, it has been proved that children do much better in the presence of a known and trusted adult unless the adult gets so overwhelmed and anxious that he or she causes the child to be even more nervous. If you can't stand to look when your child has an injection, close your eyes, but try to help with his or her emotions instead of indulging your own. If a toddler is having blood drawn and his mother begins to sob, she is not providing the strength her son needs to cope with the procedure.

A mother recently told me about when her five-year-old son was in the hospital for a tonsillectomy and how the doctor picked him up out of his bed to take him to the surgical suite.

"Ricky screamed 'Mom!' all the way down the hall until they disappeared around the corner. The doctor later said that he was well behaved once I was out of sight."

Ricky probably stopped yelling because, without his mother, he gave up hope. It's human nature. As long as someone who cares is there to listen, you'll scream. But if you think no one cares, you may stop. That does not mean you suffer less; in fact, you probably suffer more. When children have to be sedated for surgery, it is very important that parents stay with them until they fall asleep. Your child should not be carted off kicking and screaming. And after the operation, ideally you should be there when your child wakes up to provide reassurance.

Many years ago I worked next to a clinic in which children with leukemia were being treated. These children had to have repeated bone-marrow punctures—at the time, an extremely painful procedure. When I heard the children screaming during the procedure, I was moved to find out what was going on. I talked to the kids and their parents and learned that they had to come in every three weeks for the treatment. One parent said,

"Having leukemia is terrible, but these bone marrows are the worst part of it. We don't sleep the night before and our son doesn't sleep either. He gets really scared and they don't allow us to stay with him."

One day, I couldn't stand it anymore and worked up the courage to go to the front desk. I introduced myself to the doctor and asked if I could come in and help. I wasn't very welcome. They felt they were doing all they could and that I was meddling, but they finally decided to let me give it a try. I went into one of the treatment rooms where a seven-year-old girl, Sarah, was screaming her heart out while being held down by four buxom nurses.

"Have you tried having her mother stay with her?" I asked.

"Are you crazy, that would only make it worse!" one of the nurses responded. So I asked whether they would let me try to help and they reluctantly agreed. To Sarah, I said,

> *"I know you are very scared. You may not be able to do this, but if I brought your mom back in and she was right here, and you could hold her hand, would you be able to lie still? Then they wouldn't have to hold you down. You have to understand, they will only let me try it once. And if you get even more upset, then we will have to hold you down because you need to have the procedure."*

To everyone's amazement, it worked. Sarah's mother came in, sat down next to her and held her hand. Although the procedure was no different, Sarah was able to cooperate without screaming and did not need to be held down. Fortunately, we have learned a great deal more about pain relief and sedation since then. But while bone-marrow punctures and other invasive procedures are usually not as uncomfortable as they used to be, they still raise anxiety and it is important to be there to provide comfort for your child.

It may seem cruel to you that for something as simple as a blood test your child's arm is strapped down to a board. Doing the procedure correctly and as quickly as possible is the main goal and takes precedence. Unfortunately, there are times when children do have to be immobilized. And sometimes babies need to be "mummied," which means using either a big blanket or a specially designed canvas wrap that looks somewhat like a papoose. This may appear awful, but these techniques will actually make the procedure hurt less. Remember that you should be there to provide comfort.

As the child gets older, different approaches become possible. Verbal explanations become more effective, the child's curiosity helps, and there is also a healthy drive to master the situation rather than rebel or submit to it

as a victim. Children of school age and above are usually highly motivated
to understand what the doctor does and will try to be brave, participate, and
not cry when something hurts. Older children cope better with more advanced notice of a doctor's visit, and they also do better on their own for
procedures and shots—as long as they know Mom or Dad is not far away.
If you think your child can handle something without being restrained, tell
the doctors and nurses. Most children do deserve one or two chances to try
to handle things on their own.

The Child as an Active Participant

It is important to include children ages five and over in their health care as
much as possible. Even very young children can often give relevant information about their symptoms. They have their own questions to ask and can
contribute to patient–physician communication in a unique way. The more
children know about their own bodies—why it's important to brush your
teeth, why it's important to eat healthy foods—the more likely they are to
develop desirable health behaviors in the future. This is even more true for
children who have health problems such as asthma or diabetes.

A child who recognizes symptoms early is able to do things that may
help prevent serious complications. For instance, when the mother in the
following scenario brings her daughter to the doctor, she finds herself corrected.

DOCTOR: *How is she taking her insulin now?*

MOTHER: *Well, she takes the NPH in the morning and the regular at
noon and at night.*

JENNIFER: *No, Mom, I don't take the regular at noon anymore.*

MOTHER: *That's right. You don't need that anymore.*

DOCTOR: *And what about her diet?*

MOTHER: *At breakfast, I can watch her carefully and make sure she
doesn't eat the things she shouldn't. Of course, during school lunch I
have no control. Then, she spends weekends with her father and I
worry because I'm not sure that he is as diligent as I am. And she and*

her father are going on vacation for a week and so I've really been worrying . . . .

JENNIFER: *I'm very careful about what I eat at school and Dad watches me all the time. I know candy is bad and I hardly eat it anymore.*

DOCTOR: *Good for you, Jennifer! Keep up the good work.*

JENNIFER: *Every once in a while when I'm with my friends I have a soda. Is that okay?*

MOTHER: *Jennifer! You didn't tell me that!*

DOCTOR: (To mother) *It's all right.*
      (To Jennifer) *It's not the best thing for you, but you seem to be managing and you deserve something every now and then.*

JENNIFER: *I'm really trying but sometimes it's hard.*

Allowing Jennifer to volunteer her side achieved a number of desirable goals during this encounter. First, it gave the doctor a more complete picture on which to base his treatment decisions. Also, in respecting her as a participant in the encounter, he made Jennifer feel comfortable in asking some of her own questions. She had been feeling guilty about drinking the soda, worrying about what her mother would do if she found out, and what the doctor would think. While enforcing the basic message, the doctor did not become judgmental and make her feel bad about her behavior, but instead enlisted her future cooperation.

Teenagers

Although younger children pose one set of challenges, adolescents require different, but also highly skilled attention. Teenagers, while they present a tough exterior and are reluctant to communicate with their doctors, are overly concerned with their bodies. They are terrified of any unusual symptoms and need a lot of reassurance. This is especially true in our health-conscious, media-saturated culture in which they are exposed to so many misconceptions and misinformation.

A teenager who is the son of friends of mine called me unexpectedly one Sunday morning from a phone booth. Would it be all right if he came over right away? I was surprised because we never had had much communication; in fact, I couldn't remember ever having a lengthy conversation with him. When he arrived, he removed his clothes and showed me an area high up on his inner thigh where he had developed swelling and redness. He was extremely anxious and embarrassed because he thought that the swelling might be a harbinger of some sexually transmitted disease. When I asked him why he hadn't called his doctor, he said,

"The doctor might find something terrible and tell my parents."

I was able to reassure him that we were dealing with nothing more serious than a superficial infection around an ingrown hair. Fortunately, his family and ours had been friends for a long time and he felt at ease in calling me, but I was still not his doctor. It is important for pediatricians or general doctors who take care of teenagers to create an open, nonjudgmental relationship so that the patients feel comfortable enough to discuss any of their worries and ask questions freely.

In the next case we look at how a young man's appearance and manner of speech revealed that he saw himself as a macho teenager who very much wanted to be viewed as tough and didn't want to admit to any weakness. Yet while the surgeon was busy writing in the chart, the patient's posture and body language indicated that he was extremely frightened of the scheduled operation.

> PATIENT: *It seems like it never—I mean, this is the first time this has ever happened to me . . . . But then I, like, you know, I kind of thought—They are gonna cut me open, cut me up, it seems like they are going to do.*

He looks up anxiously at the doctor who does not return his glance.

> PATIENT: *I mean, like, how long is the operation? About an hour?*
>
> DOCTOR: *Oh, about forty-five minutes. Are you worried about the surgery?*
>
> PATIENT: *I am, I mean, they are going to cut me open.*

The doctor concentrates on making notes in the patient's record.

> DOCTOR: *Well, you will be asleep.*
>
> PATIENT: *When I wake up, it is going to hurt?*
>
> DOCTOR: *Not very much. Oh, it will hurt a little. What happens is you will go to sleep. They will give some sedation to you in your line. Something which goes into your vein and puts you to sleep.*
>
> PATIENT: *Are they going to shoot me up or something?*

The idea of an IV medication does not reassure this young patient who has heard a lot about intravenous drug use. The doctor fails to comprehend the significance of this question and continues his general reassurance:

> DOCTOR: *They'll keep you asleep, and they will operate on you. When you wake up it will be all done and there will be a bandage down there. You will be a little sore for a while, but after about a day or two, you won't feel any of it.*
>
> PATIENT: *What if it hurts bad? I mean, do you think it will?*

The doctor is still writing.

> DOCTOR: *No.*
>
> PATIENT: *Well, what if it does?*
>
> DOCTOR: *The nurse will give you medicine and take care of it.*
>
> PATIENT: *I'm just sort of nervous about it, that's all.*

The doctor finishes his writeup and, without looking up, concludes,

> DOCTOR: *Well, we will talk to you about it again. You don't need to worry at all. We see lots of these. People are usually very surprised how very little pain there is associated with it. You will hardly even know that you have had the surgery.*
>
> PATIENT: *All right. But it just worries me a lot.*

The doctor picks up the file and leaves the room. Even after the doctor is gone, the patient twirled around on his chair and continued to be restless and jumpy.

The doctor intended to be reassuring throughout the interview, but he never established eye contact and did not perceive the mounting anxiety in his patient. There was no sign that the adolescent relaxed after the visit and the doctor remained completely unaware. Our research nurse, noticing how upset he was, asked him a few simple questions. She found out that there were two major reasons for his anxiety. One was that the surgical procedure might damage one of his testes and therefore he would not be able to function sexually as a normal adult male. In addition, he had had an uncle who bled to death on the operating table. Small wonder he was scared! The young man had made a sincere effort to let the doctor know how frightened and scared he was. Had he been a little less so and more courageous, he might have tried to insist on answers to his underlying concerns.

Teenagers tend to do better on their own without the interference of a parent accompanying them into the examination room This allows them to communicate directly with their doctors. But it may not always be easy for them. What you, as a parent, can do is to encourage your teenager to make sure his or her questions and concerns have been heard. Before the visit, take some time to talk about how important it is not to hesitate to let the doctor know their feelings for fear of seeming cowardly or weak. Another important reason teenagers are sometimes reluctant to be honest is that they worry that parents or doctors will not keep what they are told in strict confidence. Therefore, parents and doctors themselves need to reassure adolescents that their confidences will not be betrayed.

Under very special circumstances, parents may have to be more directly involved because a physician cannot, in good conscience, keep information from those who are responsible for the patient. This applies when a physician feels there is a threat to the safety of the patient or others, as in the case of diseases that can be transmitted or suicide threats. Here's how I approach my adolescent patients:

> "I will keep everything private that you tell me unless there is something that I feel, for the sake of yourself or someone else, needs to be known to your parents. But, I will never tell them without warning you first."

The general rule of thumb is that physicians try to maintain confidentiality at all costs. If they discover something that is alarming, the first step is to encourage the patient to discuss it with his or her parents. If the teenager feels diffident about that, the doctor should suggest a family conference between the teenager, the parents, and the physician. That way, the patient does not have to face the parents alone.

Choosing a Pediatrician

"My pediatrician doesn't even like me. When I take my child in, he just tells me not to worry. I never get answers to my questions."

Even though this same kind of disappointment is voiced by patients after many other types of medical visits, a visit to the pediatrician poses its own set of unique stresses. For one thing, the parent who accompanies the child, usually the mother, is not the primary focus of the visit. The doctor's attention is divided, so it is not unusual for the parent to feel left out and poorly understood.

When young physicians are asked why they chose to go into pediatrics, many respond,

"Because I love kids."

But they also complain,

"It's the parents who are the problem."

In fact, at least 60 percent of a pediatrician's time is spent talking to parents and, it is hoped, listening to them. Yet they often think of that time as an unwelcome distraction while they enjoy the time they spend interacting with children. In our many videotaped encounters, even the doctors' tone of voice was dramatically more friendly when addressing children than when talking with adults. No wonder parents often feel left out and disappointed.

Young children are rarely able to voice their own concerns:

"I've been having a temperature every night for the past three days."
"I don't eat enough of my vegetables."
"I don't like to sleep."

Their parents need to do this for them, which makes for complex situations in the consultation room.

In choosing a pediatrician, it is a good idea to find out what his or her attitudes are toward parents. You might be tempted to ask,

"Do you hate parents too?"

But of course you can't do that. You can ask other questions about child rearing and health issues that will give you an idea. If, for example, you ask,

"What should I do—I don't seem to have enough breast milk for the baby?"

and the doctor becomes impatient and gives a judgmental reply like,

"Basically every mother can breast feed if she is really motivated; you just have to try harder,"

then you realize that your concerns, feelings of inadequacy, and fatigue are not being considered.

In this sort of situation, instead of accepting the putdown, try to engage the doctor in a dialogue. Are you a working mother? Watch the doctor's expression when you say that you need to go back to work and will be putting your child in day care. If you are lucky and your pediatrician is parent-centered as well as child-centered, you may be given helpful pointers about finding the right day-care facility, but, if not, you might simply be written off as being a bad mother. Or, if you and your child's father have a disagreement about some aspect of care, such as letting the baby cry instead of picking him up, does the doctor quickly take sides or does he listen to both of you? A family-centered pediatrician would listen. During the first few visits or perhaps even in the first encounter, you should be able to form an impression of whether you and your family will be able to work effectively with the doctor.

The setup in the doctor's office and the attitudes of the staff are also important. How child-centered is the doctor's office? Are there interesting toys, child-sized furniture, nice books to read aloud? And if there is a television, are the programs child-friendly? There should be evidence that someone has selected the programs with an eye to children. Is there an area set aside for them to move about? How about a diapering area? Safety proofing should be in evidence everywhere. The nurses and receptionists should be tolerant and know how to talk to children, but they should also be tolerant of *your* anxieties and questions. If the baby's bottle breaks and milk spills all over you, do they come to help or grumble? The pediatrician's office is the one place where everyone should expect and accept the inevitable inconveniences of being around babies and children, and you should always feel comfortable.

When Children Go to the Hospital

"Mom, I don't want to go to the hospital."
"I want to stay home with you and dad."
"If you let me stay home, I'll be good and stay in bed."

Hospitalization is even more stressful for children than adults. How would you feel if you were suddenly instructed that you needed to go to the hospital immediately? For instance, if you got a call from the doctor's office saying, *"Having reviewed your biopsy, we better put you in the hospital right away"*?

So, if you think of a young child whose comprehension is limited, who has a poorly established sense of self and reality, who has anxieties that are much more dramatic, and whose thinking is magical and unrealistic, it's not hard to imagine that such an experience would be absolutely terrifying. Children have a hard time understanding adult conversation and certainly don't know "med-speak." There are many anecdotes about the gross misunderstandings children have suffered in the hospital. A small boy heard his doctor saying,

"We'll keep him here until the fever is down."

but all he heard was,

"We'll keep him."

and he thought that that was forever. His mother found him sobbing in bed when she came to visit. There's another famous story about a child who had a swollen abdomen and heard the doctor say,

"He has edema of the belly."

He later told his mother,

"The doctor said I have a demon in my belly!"

Once in the hospital, children don't like anything about it. They are placed in strange beds that may have confining bars or covers over the top, making them feel caged in. They are awakened early and frequently, sometimes for painful procedures, given big trays of food that they may not like, and are cared for by strangers garbed in scary clothes—white coats, masks and gowns, scrub suits and surgical hats, nursing uniforms. As many as 100 people walk into a four-bed patient room in a day: doctors, interns, nursing staff, nursing aids, lab technicians, food management, cleaning personnel. Since some of these people do perform painful procedures, it is only natural that a child becomes frightened each time a new person enters the room.

The whole family gets anxious when a child goes to the hospital, and some parents tend to feel guilty, as if they, somehow, have failed. Years ago, when I held a series of group discussions for the parents of sick children, one of the topics that came up repeatedly was that, sooner or later, they blamed themselves for their child's illness. No matter what these parents had been told about the cause of the illness, they tended to think it had been brought on by something they themselves had done or failed to do. If a child was diabetic, for instance, the parents often thought they had fed him too many sweets. If a child had kidney trouble, the parents chastised themselves for allowing their baby to sit out in the cold for too long. Sometimes parents even thought the cause was psychological. When a new baby arrived in a family, for instance, and an elder child subsequently became ill, the parents assumed that the illness was their fault. They had not spent as much time with the older child since the birth of the baby and therefore felt that this "neglect" had been the cause. You, as a parent, may find yourself wondering,

What is it that I did?

What is it that I didn't do?

If I had done it differently, would my child have stayed well?

Discussing these ideas with your doctor may give you a chance to be reassured.

In addition, children tend to blame themselves when they are sick. They don't understand why it's necessary to go to the hospital, are not receptive to the reasons they need to go, and feel their parents are punishing them for something bad.

The way your child reacts to the stress of hospitalization will depend on a number of factors, especially age and stage of development. Children between one and three years old, who are in the midst of struggling for their independence, react most strongly to the restraints placed on them during hospitalization. As anyone who has observed toddlers in action knows, they are constantly trying out their newly acquired abilities: walking, running, climbing, pushing, pulling. They are learning that they can manipulate the world around them. This is a very important step in achieving autonomy. Hospitalization prevents toddlers from doing all the things that make their lives worth living. What an insult to be confined in a crib, unable to get up, and be put into diapers. Add to that the insult to a two year old who has just mastered toilet training, who will not be able to get out of bed to take care of his or her needs, perhaps even being put back in diapers again. Or the fact that a toddler may have to be fed when he has just become proud of being able to eat on his own. On the other hand, toddlers, left to their own devices, might remove IV lines or other treatments, so restraint may be needed. At these times it is especially important for the parent to be there so that the child does not feel abandoned.

Preschoolers, children between three and five, have similar reactions to separation and restraint, but at least they are better able to understand explanations from parents and caretakers. Fortunately, older children, with their increased curiosity and desire to master painful experiences, although also unhappy in the hospital, tend not to be as fundamentally threatened. When it comes to more mature children, school-aged and teenager, obviously the aspects of the hospital environment that you will be considering are very different.

An important feature to discuss with the caretaking staff is what kind of educational experience might be available and how you can help to continue what is, after all, a child's main work—namely, schooling. For adolescents, there are other considerations such as increased need for privacy and the importance of having access to their peers for support during stressful experiences. Most larger hospitals for children will have separate departments for adolescents where they have individual telephones and rooms where they can socialize. Adolescents tend to be offended when they are put in children's wards but, on the other hand, being hospitalized in the presence of adults who are very ill can also be upsetting. When all goes well, older children may later look back on hospitalization as a growth experience if they are pleased with the way they have coped on their own away from home.

Even after short hospital stays, you may notice some puzzling changes in your child's behavior. Younger infants may experience sleeping difficulties, feeding problems, and an increase in general irritability. These things often happen when a child's routine is turned upside down, disrupting the regular schedule and individual patterns of experiencing the day and night. Feeding schedules are different; it never really gets dark in a hospital room at night and there are constant noises and other things going on that are unsettling. Sometimes they show regressive behaviors—more thumb sucking, more whining, and even though the child may have been completely toilet trained before the hospital stay, accidents suddenly start happening again. Independence and recently acquired skills are the first to go when a child is really upset. If your child was just starting to speak, you may find that he's using fewer words or even baby talk. Children who were independent, outgoing, and had been gaining new skills suddenly become more clingy and dependent after a hospital stay. One parent complained to me:

"Now when I take my son to day care or if I have to go out for an evening, he raises a fuss and won't let me leave him."

Some children actually get angry at their parents after they have been in the hospital. A mother told me how upset she was when her five-year-old son, who was hospitalized to have his tonsils removed, woke up after the surgery and said,

"Go away, Mom, leave me alone."

Children may feel that you should not have allowed them to be submitted to the experience—you somehow should have protected them. If your child withdraws and turns away instead of greeting you enthusiastically, don't take it personally; it really is a compliment. It means you were missed so much that you will not be immediately forgiven.

Preparing

As soon as the determination is made that your child needs to go to the hospital, it is a good idea to find out from the doctor as much as you can about what will be involved. If your child is old enough, ask the doctor to explain what is going to happen. For many children, it is reassuring to know that not only will their parent be with them, but, in fact, their own doctor will come and see them to provide continuity with someone they trust.

Children are all too familiar with hospitals through television. Unfortunately, in the media, patients are always shown in crisis—bleeding to death, having CPR, relatives bursting into tears. Recently I heard that one of my patients, a little girl, when informed that her favorite uncle had died, promptly asked, *"Who shot him?"* It never occurred to her that he might have died a natural death. Children are no strangers to violent death and drastic illness, so it is very important to explain that, in real life, hospitals are not only for people who are very sick, but are also there to take care of you and make you better.

When your doctor tells you where your child is going to be admitted, ask some questions: Are there pre-admission tours for children? Quite a few hospitals will schedule visits for children beforehand so they can get acquainted and walk through the wards, learn where they will sleep, and see other children. Some will even show the operating room, the recovery room, and the whole surgical suite. This is often helpful to older children because it demystifies the unknown. On the other hand, you know your child best; if you think he or she is going to be more scared by seeing all the strange places with all the instruments and the dramatic medical equipment, then you may not choose to do that part.

Does the hospital have a playroom? Be sure to ask about the availability of a play area. One little girl I take care of who had been hospitalized many times told me,

> "When I go to the hospital, it's not like you're being punished or something. They don't lock you up. You meet a lot of nice doctors and nurses and they let you go to the playroom and everything."

The playroom is often the one thing that makes a hospital tolerable for children. One of the ground rules there is that doctors and nurses are not allowed to perform any painful procedures, so it's a "safe" area. When I visit the children's ward in the morning, I see the children waiting anxiously at the playroom door, asking when it's going to open. With its child-sized furnishings and decorations, toys and easels, it's part of a child's world and a place where they feel comfortable. There is always a doctor's corner with medical equipment that gives children a chance to apply bandages, listen with a stethoscope, pretend they are giving injections, and even "operate." They invariably want to be the doctor or the nurse, but not the patient; it's their chance to take charge and, in so doing, master the experience. They are also encouraged to make paintings and write poetry, which helps them and yields interesting insights into their perceptions of what is going on.

It's important to understand which aspects of the experience are going to be the toughest for your child. The ideas that you need to keep in mind are not different from those you would use to prepare your child for any difficult experience. You should be truthful and careful in the timing of your preparation so that younger children don't worry too long and older ones have time to begin to get themselves ready mentally and physically. If you have an idea of what exactly will happen in the hospital, it's important to talk about it with your child. There are helpful books for children that deal not only with the hospital in general, but also with particular experiences of children who undergo surgery or illness.

In addition, focus your own energies on making the experience a better one for your child and you. Under optimal circumstances, with good preparation, the whole family mobilized for support, and a sensitive treatment team, the experience may even have positive aspects. When the family has weathered the stress and especially when the child has gotten through it in good shape, there is a sense of accomplishment, a feeling of *We as a family can handle tough situations.*

When You and Your Child Get There

As soon as possible after your child has been admitted, interpret his or her needs to the nursing staff—food likes and dislikes, allergies, or personal habits. In most hospitals, the nurse will ask questions about what words your child uses for certain functions as well as preferences and dislikes so as to make the hospital experience as similar to home as possible.

Ask the charge nurse about general policies, not only visiting hours that you hope will be unlimited, but also about any other ground rules: Are brothers and sisters allowed to visit? How many visitors at a time? What are you allowed to bring in? If your child loves tacos, is it all right to bring him one? Unless you ask, you may not realize, for instance, that some balloons have been found to be dangerous and most hospitals won't allow you to bring them.

Once you know when you can visit, it will help your child to have you there as much as possible. It has consistently been shown that children whose parents have been able to stay with them while they were in the hospital really do a great deal better. However, some parents tell us that they find visiting difficult. They really don't know what to do and feel out of their element. Although they have every intention of providing reassurance, it can be difficult because of the stress they themselves are experiencing. And the more children see that their parents are anxious, the more upset they tend to become. Make an effort not to let your own distress show too much in front of your child. Get up your courage so that you can be a source of strength and support. Nothing is more unsettling to a child than to see a parent "lose it." If something painful and difficult is being done and you go to pieces, it will make it more difficult for your child. Try to keep your cool. Your child relies on your strength for help through difficult experiences and has to be able to count on you.

Make a plan for the visit. You know your child. He or she probably doesn't want you to sit beside the bed and start a serious conversation. Parents and their children rarely engage in long, one-on-one conversations at home—and, if so, it often means there is a problem to discuss! At home, there are a great many things that parents and children do together: shopping, working in the kitchen and garden, playing. In the hospital, however, when parents come to visit they may feel uneasy because they don't quite know what to do and neither does the child.

Bring a favorite game, a book—use the time well. Try to think of things to keep your child occupied while you are not there. Does she like to do hairdos on Barbie dolls? Does he want a Lego set to build a fancy truck? If possible, bring other family members. There's nothing wrong with calling in reinforcements. If the hospital allows it, siblings are a great distraction; children who seem miserable suddenly perk up when a sibling comes in. Just as in the playroom, you may be surprised that your child, who was listless a minute ago, seems a lot better.

One young patient of mine, Jason, was born with abnormalities of his bladder and his entire urinary tract. He had to undergo many operations, but despite all this, he was extremely well adapted throughout his illness. Now, as an adolescent, he is a delightful young person who is a good student, has earned a black belt in karate, and is even a good surfer. When I asked his mother why she thought he had done so well throughout the experience, one of the things she mentioned was,

> *"We always stayed with him . . . every surgery, every hospitalization, and whenever anything that was difficult for him had to be done."*

Jason had to adapt to a great many difficult restrictions and undergo many frightening procedures, but his parents were ever responsive to his needs, very empathetic, and were always truthful with him. For instance, in this next interview Jason's father talks about what he did when Jason's preschool discharged him because of his special needs.

> FATHER: *Preschool situation was good for the boy—Jason loved it. But the teachers felt uncomfortable with him being there. So they asked us to remove him from the preschool. He loved it there. It was difficult to explain why they would not accept him. And why a teacher would not accept him in class.*
>
> *I told him the truth in a nice way. That for him, sometimes there are going to be some things that we are going to have to deal with individually . . . . We spent a lot of time on his self-esteem and for him to not think that it was his fault.*

Throughout the experience, his mother was also very sensitive to his distress and his unique reactions. Years after the actual event, she told me, with tears in her eyes:

MOTHER: *The hardest things were times when he'd come to me and say, "Mom, why can't I go to the bathroom like everybody else? I want to stand up." And his being only three years old and so innocent, for me, as a mother, it was pretty heartbreaking. He wanted to be like the other children. That was hard.*

This mother was always responsive to her child's concerns. After one of his surgeries, Jason no longer had a belly button. Although he was motivated to go swimming with the other children, he was embarrassed when he had to put on a bathing suit. As his mother told us,

"He wanted a belly button, which he didn't have, and that was hard because in the summer the kids would tease him. They'd say, 'Well, you don't have a belly button!' When you are four years old, a belly button is a very important thing to have along with your bathing suit."

So during another one of his major surgeries, his parents made special arrangements to have a plastic surgeon come in to make him a new belly button—that was his Christmas present! This extra procedure went way beyond the call of duty and demonstrates that empathetic parents and a responsive surgeon were able to help a young child deal with one of his concerns.

Another remarkable thing is that when a child has an overwhelming abnormality or serious condition, caretakers are usually not as responsive to what seem like small side issues on the part of the patient. One of the dehumanizing aspects of illness is that decisions are made for you on the basis of other people's value systems, not on your preferences. A surgeon might have said,

"He's lucky to be alive! We're reconstructing his whole urinary tract and intestinal tract. It's silly to even think about a belly button!"

But in this case, they responded to his individual concerns instead of making a medically driven decision about what was or was not important for him.

Every child who has an illness responds differently and you, as a parent, are the one who best knows what is important. Therefore, find out specifically what your child minds about the illness and treatment, no matter how trivial it seems, and respond. Sometimes you can't do anything, but at least you can provide reassurance,

> *"I understand why not having a belly button makes you feel funny. We'll see what we can do about it."*

Whether or not it's possible to adapt the treatment or procedure, at least you will be in a better position to understand instead of getting angry at your child.

One of the things children, like all of us, are most afraid of when they go to the doctor or hospital is pain. This needs to be accepted and realized. It's infuriating to hear a nurse or doctor say to your child:

> *"It really doesn't hurt that much,"*

when you can see that it really does. The nurse is not going to know how much it hurts; the only one who knows is your child and you've got to help get it across. There are ways of helping your child tell you how much it hurts. Charts that allow children to point to a picture or a number help them in describing their pain. In any case, the first step is for you and the staff to acknowledge your child's pain and to do something about it.

Once you feel that a serious attempt has been made to assess the level of pain, find out what options are available. What can be done to make your child more comfortable? When it comes to injections, blood drawing, and minor procedures such as sewing up superficial skin wounds, there are local sprays and other measures that can be helpful in preventing pain. For example, when applied ahead of time locally to the skin, EMLA® Creme has proven very effective. If the hospital staff is reluctant to give your child medication for pain, you need to understand that there may be times when medication is dangerous. Sedatives and painkillers may mask important symptoms and some medications can cause unsafe side effects.

Of course, besides the actual physical pain of an injection, there also tends to be a lot of anxiety that is a significant part of the "pain." The very idea of being stuck with a needle can cause grown men to fall into a dead faint. Early in my career, I was part of a program that involved the routine drawing of blood from a large number of able-bodied young military recruits. On one occasion, several lines formed and, in charge of one of them, I drew blood from the first soldier without difficulty. But as I inserted a needle into the second soldier, the third one, who was standing in line and watching, fainted away. For several moments, this big, macho recruit lay motionless on the ground. Everyone assumed that I had done something terrible to him. Having observed this, one by one, all the recruits in my line moved over to another line amid murmurs of,

"I don't want her to take my blood!"

There are also behavioral ways of dealing with pain. A technique called "imaging" helps children imagine favorite places and activities while undergoing painful procedures. And because children have such a vivid imagination, they are very responsive to hypnosis. They live much of their lives in fantasy, so it's not as hard for them to escape reality.

One of my patients, a teenager named Cheryl, suffered a lot of pain from complications related to kidney dialysis. The treatment team had a terrible time finding ways to give her relief. Her mother told me that she had heard about a famous Hollywood hypnotist who "could do wonders" and whom she wanted to help her daughter. She was known as Pat Collins, "The Hip Hypnotist." There was nothing to lose; it wasn't dangerous, and if she could help, I was willing to try anything. So I invited Ms. Collins to see Cheryl, which, at the time, caused quite a sensation in our conservative hospital. The administration made it clear that I would be held fully responsible for anything that happened.

She arrived, a flamboyant blonde wearing a long black dress. Her makeup was heavy and somewhat vampire-like. Activity in the halls came to a halt as staff and patients stopped to stare. She swept into the dialysis unit with me and I introduced her to my patient. Cheryl was anxious about the upcoming procedure, but she turned out to be a very good hypnotic subject and her pain was greatly reduced.

What was even more important was that Ms. Collins subsequently taught Cheryl self-hypnosis so that she could deal with the pain on her own. How much of the success of this entire experience was due to the fact that here was a person who really recognized and accepted Cheryl's suffering, and who came across strongly as being there to help her, and how much was due to the actual hypnosis is not really relevant. Even when medication is given, besides its biological effect, there is also a placebo effect. The very fact that something is being done helps patients feel better.

Has the hospital staff made decisions about your child without you?

There are bound to be important things going on while you're not even there. If, for instance, a procedure that is not an emergency is scheduled without any warning, you have a right to question how that happened, although there may be a perfectly good reason. To serve as your child's advocate, it is best to negotiate beforehand, but also to realize that there may be limits to how far you will get. If you are determined not to leave your child during a painful procedure, explain this in advance so that you don't suddenly find yourself in a face-off with someone who insists,

"No, no, no. . . . You can't be with your child."

You actually have the right to be present with your child during procedures unless your presence interferes with what has to be done. Although it seems as if an awful lot of people are making decisions, ultimately it is the doctor who will direct your child's treatment. Insist that you be involved! Hospitals are attuned to parent and patient satisfaction and want to please. Even though you may not win every inning, you will still have an impact.

You and the staff and, when possible, your child, need to work together to achieve the best results. Otherwise, you may be torn in too many directions. It is important to try to put yourself in the state of mind of the caretaking personnel. There may be times when you feel that your child is being unreasonable and the staff will need your help in setting limits. If, on the other hand, you perceive the staff as being insensitive, then you will need to be more protective and supportive of your child. Even though it may be tough at times, make a sincere effort to work with the staff because if they see you as an adversary, it won't help. Basically, you, the doctors, and nurses are a team in wanting to help your child get well. And it is only human that the professionals will knock themselves out for families whom they see as cooperative.

Establishing Future Habits

The children and young people who are visiting the pediatrician today are going to be the adults who will set the tone for health care and behavior in the next century. That is why it is important now to promote positive attitudes toward health and medical care in the hope that the next generation will enjoy good health and take better care of themselves. Although this is not easy to achieve, parents and caregivers should work together in stressing that a visit to the doctor is not a necessary evil but a privilege. Almost all of us dread visiting the doctor and dentist, and children are quick to pick up on it. Good behavior and positive attitudes need to be modeled by adults to make the experience of medical care as positive as possible and minimize anxiety and discomfort. *"Do as I say and not as I do"* is not an effective way of educating the young.

Does the actual conduct of a doctor in a medical visit with a child make a difference in that child's eventual attitudes about medicine and health? Most adults remember their very early visits with the doctor. I have been impressed by how, when asked to reflect on their own childhood experiences, many are able to recall early visits to the pediatrician or dentist with specific details. I hear about tremendous fears and am told too many horror stories. But I also hear about positive experiences that certain individuals had during their formative years. In fact, young pediatricians often describe how impressed they were with their family pediatrician during their own childhood. They saw the doctor as an admirable role model who inspired them to choose a medical career. We have already come a long way, but we still do have quite a distance to go in making people's attitudes about medical care more positive. Children's issues, and the importance of being sensitive and responsive in providing health care for them, are all too often minimized:

> *"What's the difference, life is tough and children have to get used to it. Everybody has to go through stresses and, in the long run, it may be good for children to have stressful experiences."*

Preventing these stresses from becoming overwhelming and helping children to cope better is essential. In the interest of promoting positive attitudes toward health care in adults, we must invest in children. Making that investment is eminently justified, for, after all, they are our future.

THE HOSPITAL

▼
▼

Mrs. X, a new member of the board of directors of a leading New York hospital, arrived for her first meeting. She was not sure which entrance to use, so she decided to try the one nearest to where she had parked. Little did she know that she had entered the OB-GYN pavilion, urgent care. At the front desk, she was greeted by a hospital staff member who requested identifying information. Shortly afterwards a nurse appeared, told her they were ready for her, and ushered her into another area. Before she knew what happened, she found herself in an examination room with her feet up in stirrups!

Being Admitted

Although this story may have been embellished in repeated telling, it is true. Being admitted to the hospital is like finding yourself on a conveyor belt being whisked away into a sterile land of uncertainty and fear. Just locating the right parking space and the proper entrance can be daunting. Having to pass by guards and produce identification is not the warmest welcome either. *"I felt like a criminal, as if they expected I had a gun hidden somewhere,"* one conservatively dressed, mild-mannered visitor told me. This whole ritual can make you sense that they are trying to keep you out instead of helping you in. Almost no concessions are made to the fact that patients feel anxious, uncomfortable, and alienated.

You are greeted by a deluge of paperwork and everyone keeps instructing you to "sign here." It seems as if your insurance status and financial position are all that matter. No one seems to care about why you're there or how you're feeling For you it's a big moment—

"My God, I'm going to the hospital!"

For them, it's—

"Here's another patient to process for admission."

Then a wheelchair arrives with someone assigned to push you, even though you may be perfectly capable of walking. While you desperately clutch the personal possessions piled awkwardly in your lap, an attendant wheels you up one corridor and down another, into and out of elevators. It's not uncommon for patients to lose their sense of direction, leaving them feeling completely disoriented. Family or friends may not be able to accompany patients while they are being taken up to their rooms because they are parking the car or attending to other practical details. By the time your family starts looking for you, you have already been delivered to the room and are convinced you will never be reunited with them.

While you are settling in, you are asked to relinquish your valuables for "safe-keeping." Safe from what? Will someone really try to take them while you are asleep? This makes patients feel as if they are in hostile territory and that they have no control. If you can't keep your watch in your bedside table for fear someone is going to take it, how safe will *you* be? Even though this policy is ultimately for patients' benefit, it makes them feel even further stripped of their individuality and causes them to lose trust. Without your wristwatch and wallet, without identification and credit cards, who are you? Without a word of explanation, a staff member fastens a plastic identification bracelet around your wrist. Your name is there on the little white adhesive tag. Now you are completely packaged and labeled. The staff look at it before looking at you. Would they know who you were without it? You begin to feel like a nobody, that no one knows where you are, that no one really cares.

Hospitalization can be devastating. Even under the best circumstances, it has consistently been reported as dehumanizing because the hospital presents insurmountable obstacles to communication. All the elements that normally make communication difficult between doctors and patients become acute. At least when you go to the doctor for an office visit, you still have the option of presenting yourself as a fully dressed person able to stand up and walk out. But in the hospital, you are stripped of your independence as well as your clothes, which makes you feel as if you have no autonomy left. Flat on your back in bed and not feeling well, you are left to deal with a whole army of changing health professionals to whom you are only one of many. You may feel more like a victim and less than ever like an active partner in the health-care process.

Hospitals have always been busy places where patients have felt lost in the shuffle. Most of us are pretty well prepared by now for the fact that we're going to have to be interviewed by ten different people, give all kinds of information, and have our paperwork ready. But not everyone is able to cope. The next case illustrates what happened to one patient who was extremely respectful and too shy to challenge authority. The interview, videotaped in the mid-1960s, features Mr. Schultz, an elderly European who went to see a doctor in a hospital clinic because he had been having some abdominal symptoms. He had to undergo a number of tests and was asked to come back in a week. On this next visit, when he was told that his condition was sufficiently serious to require admission (many patients don't realize that the word "admit" means hospitalize), he completely failed to understand what was happening to him:

> *"Well, after a week I went back again and she asked me, 'How do you feel now?' "*
> *"I feel pretty good, I said."*
> *" 'Let me have some of your specimen,' she said."*
> *"Well, I did. Evidently they analyzed it. They know all about it, <u>but I didn't</u>. I came to the conclusion by myself. Then she said, 'I'm all through with you now. You're feeling pretty good you say? Now you go over to office SoAndSo, to desk SoAndSo, suchandsuch number.' "*

Although Mr. Schultz didn't know it, he was going through the various steps required for hospital admission. The next thing he knew, he was told to remove his clothes.

"*Well, I went over there, they checked up, they gave me the papers to go along with it.*

'Why don't you just sit down and there will be somebody here for you,' they said. Oh, after an hour or so, finally an attendant comes over, a lady, with a wheelchair.

'Is your name Schultz?' she asked me.

'Yes, Ms.,' I answered.

'Here's a paper bag, here's your pajamas, and you just take your clothes off, put it all in a paper bag' she told me."

At this point, he still did not realize that he was being hospitalized:

"*I didn't know what was going on.*

'Tell me, what's going on here?' I said.

'I don't know,' she answered."

His interpretation was that staff wasn't allowed to give that information to patients. He told us,

"*I know that much. They're not supposed to talk about it.*"

He was put in a wheelchair, pushed to a ward, and put in a bed. It was a week before he understood why this was happening to him.

"*What was so mysterious to me was that it went on for a whole week. After that, every other day, the doctor comes in, he was awful busy, I could see that.*

I was all right. I wasn't lonely. I didn't have pain. I was all right. But I was kind of worried about <u>why I was there</u>.

So after a week, the doctor came around. Oh yes, the doctor usually brought in some students . . . . I shouldn't say students. Outside doctors. They donate time and skill, so I was told later on. There were five or six of them. They go from bed to bed. Ask a question, see what's the matter. And I suppose, they take their choice, if they want to search beyond it, or whatever they are going to do.

So I understood that, not that I was told or I knew about it.

The doctor told me: 'You have something in there and I don't like that. I don't like that at all. That ought to come out.'"

> *Oh, I said. He was busy and he said he'd see about it and he walked away. I was still in a daze."*

Mr. Schultz consistently defended any behavior on the part of the doctors that might have been uncomfortable for him or even incomprehensible. He needed to hold them in the highest respect because they were the authorities on whom he was completely dependent.

> *"I didn't know what was going on. He was a good man. A very good doctor. Although he never talked with me much . . . .*
>
> *He finally came after I was there for two weeks. I must say, I steadily was going down. The doctor came near me, near the bed. He stood there and rubbed his chin. . . . I know he was worrying. I looked at him.*
>
> *'How do you feel?' he asked me.*
>
> *'All right, Doc.' I could hardly speak anymore. But you know what? I figured it was the end. So what? The doctor said to me,*
>
> *'I want to talk to you but I haven't got the time right now but I'll be back in fifteen or twenty minutes,' the doctor said to me. He went away and came back in fifteen minutes. Then he sat down on the bed, which he had never done with any other patient.*
>
> *'Well, I have to tell you something,' he said to me. 'You're an older man than I am . . . .'"*

This was the only time the doctor recognized Mr. Schultz as a person in a positive way.

Schultz continues,

> *'I'll put it bluntly to you. I think you can take it. You have a tumor in the rectum. It has to come out. There's two ways about it. You can get operated on. Or you can live with your tumor. It's up to you. If you decide to live with your tumor, I guarantee you, we do the best for you, you get the best treatment, but I'm sorry I have to tell you that you won't last long. It's in the last stage.'*
>
> *'Oh,' I said.*
>
> *Then he got up from the bed, stood there, and said, 'The other way, there's going to be surgery.'*

If there was any surgery necessary, I was going to ask him if he would be present if some other doctor operated on me. It seems like he must have been a mind reader as well as a good surgeon. He said, 'I can't hold you any longer in the condition you're in. Something has to be done. So, it's up to you now.'

'Doc . . .' I said, 'Surgery.' I didn't care what happened. I didn't care.

'Very well,' he replied, 'tomorrow morning, 7 o'clock, you're going in for surgery.'

I opened my mouth, I was going to ask him. But I thought, "No, I'm not a kid anymore." It would be like a kid, if I were to ask that question.

But he turned around and he said, 'And <u>I'm</u> going to do the surgery.' That's when I came to life!" (Claps his hands.)

Obviously, this is an extreme case. This patient was a modest, nondemanding elderly man who submitted to whatever needed to be done and accepted the attention most gratefully. He hardly interacted with any of the caretaking personnel. Worst of all, he had to wait three weeks before one individual physician finally engaged in a direct dialogue with him.

Although few patients discover themselves on a hospital ward without any understanding of why they are there, many do find themselves feeling helpless. One of my projects involved studying ward rounds at a county hospital. Among the questions we asked patients was,

"Do you understand why you are here?"

Their answers revealed that many had only a vague idea:

"I'm sick . . . ."
"I'm going to have an operation."
"The doctor said I had to come in."

Many of them were not highly educated and, for some, English was not their first language. Although that factor might have contributed, even patients with better understanding may experience a surprising degree of confusion about important matters.

In order to get yourself oriented and take charge from the moment you are admitted, it's imperative to get as much information as you can. Also remember that throughout the experience, you do have the right to question, *not* to sign, and to refuse. For instance, if you are given a surgical consent form to sign at the time of admission and there are complications mentioned that you did not anticipate, you should request to talk directly to the surgeon before signing. You have every right and every responsibility to question anything you don't understand or that you feel may be unacceptable. Patients who are sick and feel dependent are afraid of annoying the doctor and staff. It is true that if you do refuse to sign a form, you may actually get a very negative response. Don't be surprised if the person handling the form says something to the tune of,

"If you aren't ready to have the surgery done, why didn't you say so before? Now you're here and we're all ready to proceed and you suddenly say No."

But it's not your fault if you weren't completely informed before. Here is where a patient's "backbone" is essential. Assert yourself!

Being There

One of the many demeaning, dehumanizing aspects of being in the hospital is that some of the private things in our lives suddenly become public concern. You have to ask for embarrassing services from strangers—help with an annoying itch under your plaster cast, assistance to get to the bathroom or, worse yet, a bedpan. You are questioned about details that you would rather not discuss, such as whether you wear false teeth or have had a bowel movement. When you leave your room to venture out into the highly trafficked corridor, it's not in clothing, but in a scanty gown open at the back. And it seems that, unfailingly, the doctor comes to see you when you haven't had a chance to wash your face or comb your hair. You know that you are looking your worst. It's only natural that you would feel embarrassed in these situations, but remember that you are not the only one. The hospital is an environment where no one expects you to be at your best.

Patients can actually make things worse by trying to avoid embarrassment. Let's say that you are supposed to go to X ray wearing that inadequate little hospital gown, but you decide to wear something of your own because it makes you feel more comfortable and covers you up better. Then when you arrive at X ray, you are told that you must undress and put on a hospital gown. By trying to adapt the environment to your personal preferences, you have only created new complications because now you have to undress in a place where there may be no privacy. So, in some situations, the best advice is to grin and bear it. While many of the inconveniences in the hospital are not negotiable, understanding them may help you to accept them.

Until you are hospitalized, you may not realize that a hospital room is really not a comfortable place to be sick, to rest, or to recover. Will your insurance pay for a private or semi-private room? Patients who are alone sometimes feel isolated and even fearful that there will be no one there if they need help, but semi-private rooms are not always easy either. Roommates argue over the television—one wants to watch football, the other likes PBS. One prefers the volume low, the other high. Patients who do share a room may worry about what to do if the person in the next bed needs help.

The temperature can be arctic and extra blankets may be hard to wangle. All day and all night there is nonstop noise pollution: unintelligible pages over the speaker system, doctors are called, bells ring, IV monitors sound alarms, myriad mysterious beeps and other computerized sounds. Why is the door always open? You can hear other patients calling out in need of help. When you hear people sounding miserable, you tend to agonize along with them.

When patient satisfaction questionnaires were handed out at a major hospital, one elderly patient's response indicated that everything had been fine, but that there was one thing she thought was insensitive. Every once in a while, a voice came over the public address system saying,

"Room 237, the end is near . . . Room 237, the end is near."

What the voice was really saying was,

"Room 237, eng-in-eer,"

but in her anxiety she misinterpreted it!

It may seem to you as if hospital routines are planned exclusively for the doctors and hospital staff, not for patients. You may begin to feel like a guinea pig with all the tests and procedures that you are subjected to. Although it may not appear that way, they are probably necessary for you to receive the best treatment or to check your progress.

Nurses wake you up in the dark at five in the morning when you've just finally drifted off after a sleepless night. *"Good Morning!"* and a thermometer is stuck in your mouth, a tourniquet is wrapped around your arm, and you feel the sting of a needle. Certainly while you're sick, you have a hard enough time sleeping. Then when somebody comes in when it's still dark and wakes you up, it seems like deliberate sadism. Why can't the morning routines take place later?

In an ideal world, everything would be planned around the patient. But in the hospital hundreds of professionals are expected to do certain tasks; surgeons make their rounds early because they have to be in the operating room before 8, nurses start waking up patients at 5 A.M. because their reports must be finished both for the doctors and the shift change. Nursing shifts change at 7 A.M. in many hospitals. The night nurse has to report on her patients' conditions to the morning nurse who comes on duty next. If there is blood to be drawn, it must be done early enough so that the doctor will have the results by the time he or she visits. Did the blood pressure change during the night? Did the patient's temperature go up? Was the patient able to take the medication? A complete report is handed over to the next shift. In order to do that for a large group of patients, nurses must start early.

Even though you are surrounded by so many people, you feel alone, isolated, and poorly understood. All day long, an assortment of well-intentioned people, from the chief surgeon to the window washer, parade through the room all asking the same question: *"Are you feeling better today?"* For patients with special needs, this can be even tougher. One elderly patient who was blind told us that the hospital staff would continue to give her written material:

"Here's the menu, pick out your supper,"

and she'd say,

"But, you know, I am blind, I can't read."

Or they'd come in and say, *"This is the consent form you have to sign for the next surgery,"* and she would again remind them, *"I'm blind, I cannot see."* And of course she resented having to say this over and over. Her blindness was clearly indicated on her chart and there was an obvious notice over her bed to inform caretakers.

A young woman was appalled by the lack of human sympathetic response on the part of the staff to her physical limitations. Years earlier, she had been paralyzed from the waist down in a skating accident. Her present admission was for the surgical repair of her urinary tract. Each time the surgeon made his daily rounds, he said,

"Why aren't you up and about—it's better for you to walk!"

In each instance, she replied,

"I can't walk, I'm paralyzed."

Besides being offended, she was also frightened that her postoperative care might not be optimal because the doctor continued to be unaware of her underlying medical problem.

"If he doesn't know I'm paralyzed, that the circulation in my legs is obviously not good, and that I have no sensation in the lower part of my body," she said to me, *"won't that make a difference in the way he will care for me?"*

Patients frequently complain that they are transported to different parts of the hospital for various procedures and then are left stranded. The volunteer who took you to X ray in a wheel chair, for instance, disappears, leaving you abandoned. Even though you know you can walk, you are expected to wait for the chair. You feel like an invalid and know you are dependent on the staff. Therefore, it is always worth the effort to create alliances with those involved in your care. Instead of being silent while a caretaker is attending to you, attempt brief small talk that will help establish a bond. Even if you exchange only a few words,

"I saw you here earlier this morning, you must have very long hours!"

you've made it known that you are relating to that person as one human being to another. It's very important to acknowledge the staff as fellow human beings, not just as instruments of fate. If you establish even a minimal relationship, you will be more likely to be treated like a person, and you will meet less resentment when you ask a question such as, *"How long will it be before you can take me back to my room?"*

There are so many people that it seems you never see the same one twice. The people you see most consistently may be the housekeeping personnel because they usually work a full work week every day at the same time. When you're confined to a hospital bed, it's difficult to have any idea about what's going on. If you ask a question, you are usually referred to someone else. One patient who was scheduled to have surgery made many attempts during the course of the day to get in touch with a friend who had come to be with her on the day of the operation:

> *"My friend was waiting for me outside the recovery room. In the meantime, I was lying in my bed back in my own room. They kept postponing my surgery all day long. They took me down to the operating suite twice thinking they were ready to do the surgery and each time they returned me to my room. But nobody told my friend. She was waiting hours and thinking something terrible must have happened to me. I was back in my bed, increasingly anxious and had no way of communicating."*

You are afraid to do anything out of the norm because you are so dependent. If you tell the nurse, *"I was supposed to have my pain medication at three and now it's four,"* or make other criticisms, you fear there will be retribution and no one will come the next time you ring. When you do ring the bell for medication and no one answers, you hesitate to ring it again. Finally a nurse's aid shows up, and when you tell her that you would like to see the nurse, she disappears and you lie there waiting. No one comes. Hooked up to an IV or otherwise incapacitated, you can't even get up to go to the bathroom. You've made the ultimate transition from person to patient, from independence to total dependence.

What can you do when the lines of communication break down? Selectively pick issues that you really need help with. Don't ask too many people and don't ask the same person over and over. You may get different and confusing answers or they may get tired of your questions. When a new shift starts, for instance, and you have a new nurse, you may not realize that the preceding shift has probably given her a complete report so you do not need to repeat your entire history. But be sure that they have the essentials. Inquire tactfully,

"Did the other nurse tell you that I got sick from the pain medication?"

instead of complaining,

"Don't you know that I got sick from that other medication?"

If you have a question and are told to ask someone else, find out as much as you can about when that person will be by to see you. Sometimes all you can do is discover who would be the right person to ask:

"I have a friend waiting for me downstairs who doesn't know my oper-ation was postponed. Whom should I talk to about that?"

Or, for a different scenario,

"Whom should I ask when my doctor will be here?"

Many patients have told me that they constantly feel pressured to say that they're feeling better and that they are labeled "chronic complainers" if they don't. When people keep asking, *"You're feeling better aren't you?"* it's basically because they want you to feel better and it's not easy to respond, *"No, I'm feeling worse,"* or, *"No, I don't feel any better than I did yesterday."* In the hospital, everyone wants you to smile and say, *"I'm fine! I'm better!"* That makes you think that no one truly realizes how bad you feel. You may be right because even the most empathetic health professional can never really know.

Then one day, the doctor decides it's time for you to get out of bed. You may be met with disapproval or even contempt if you show any reluc-tance to get moving. Especially when it comes to physiotherapy, you may feel that you are constantly asked to do things that you are, in fact, unable to do. Although physical therapists do seem pushy, it's part of their job—they are there to help you become active and regain your strength.

Medical scientists have learned in the past two decades that more activity, sooner, is almost always good for you. Prolonged bed rest is not. Back in the 1940s, there were a number of diseases such as rheumatic fever, nephritis, tuberculosis, and certain orthopedic conditions for which patients were put to bed for as long as a year or more in the hope that rest would promote healing. For some of these conditions, there are now specific treatments, but even for those whose treatment hasn't changed, it has been learned that not only is there no advantage in staying in bed, but that it actually retards recovery. The instances in which prolonged bed rest is actually recommended—an endangered pregnancy, for instance—are rare indeed. Most people are astonished to hear how soon patients are asked to get out of bed, even following such major procedures as open-heart surgery. Although it's important to realize that you will recover more quickly and completely if you become active as soon as possible, there may be times when you need to let the staff know that you really do not feel up to it and why.

Often health professionals demonstrate insufficient awareness of how uncomfortable a patient may be after a procedure and how long the discomfort may last. After all, every patient is different. If you think that what you are being asked to do is inappropriate, be sure to discuss it with the doctors and nurses. If, for example, you are asked to get up and walk for fifteen minutes but get tired before that, inquire if it is really essential that you be up for that length of time without taking a short rest.

In reading about all the negative aspects of being in the hospital, you may wonder how anyone can stand it. But sick people do find that there are many comforting things about being there. It's nice to think that highly trained professionals with all sorts of technical resources are right down the hall in case you need them. As much as you wanted to get home, once you are discharged and are back in your own bed, you may realize that you even miss some of the hospital's services. Patients find themselves very tired, have questions but no one to ask, and are sometimes in need of help. So while many things infringe on your privacy and independence in the hospital, and although everything isn't done to your taste and convenience, it feels good to have twenty-four-hour-a-day supervision, someone who checks on you, and someone who does things for you.

When Will the Doctor Come to See You?

It's your doctor who launched you into this experience. He was always there for you before. Now, where is he? You need him now more than ever before. So why do you feel so abandoned? You try to second guess when he will come. You know he visits every day, but you've been waiting for those precious ten minutes for the last twenty-four hours.

When the doctor finally does arrive, you may be in the bathroom or asleep. Communicating while you are flat on your back also puts you at a disadvantage. When the doctor is standing right over you, it's difficult to remember exactly what you wanted to say. The doctor's visit tends to be very short, and if you haven't had the chance to think about what to say and forget something, you may have to wait another twenty-four hours for the next visit. If you do think of something too late and ask the nurse, the typical response is,

> *"The doctor was here to see you this morning. I'm not sure we can get him to come back. If it's something really important, I can call him on the phone."*

Then you begin to wonder how important your question really was.

Since the doctor cannot be there all the time, he or she has to delegate care to a host of other doctors whom you have never seen before. And as soon as you do get to know one of them, that doctor may transfer to another department. A mother whose child was very ill told me,

> *"I was appalled the first time we had rotation of doctors. You get to be very dependent on your doctor. This is the man with the answers, this is the man you turn to. And suddenly one day you find out, he's not there. I was devastated! What do you mean he's not there?"*

How can you make the most out of the limited time you do have with your physician? Find out what time he or she is expected so that you are prepared. The nurse in charge should be able to tell you what she knows. Then, plan ahead. Before seeing your doctor, think about all the things you would like to discuss. It is a good idea to keep a notepad by the side of your bed to jot down items that you may forget when the doctor is actually standing there. Then, when your doctor arrives, you can always ask when he or she plans to come back to see you. In general, most doctors will warn you when they are not going to be available,

"While I won't be here tomorrow, Dr. SoAndSo will look in on you."

But if your doctor doesn't volunteer this information, ask who will take care of you or whom to call in an emergency. What if you forget one of the most important things you wanted to ask? If it's life or death, ask the nurse to get him back. But, in most instances, you'll find that if you discuss it with the nurse, she will be able to help.

In larger hospitals and especially teaching hospitals, doctors sometimes discuss complex surgery, serious illnesses, and treatment with one another while standing over a patient's bed. When listening to such graphic descriptions, you may tend to assume, *"They're talking about me!"* when, in fact, the discussion is probably about another case. Do physicians realize that patients, who are afraid anyway, may grossly misinterpret what they hear? The medical team often gets so task oriented, so motivated to work out a particular technical problem or to arrive at a difficult diagnosis that they forget that a patient is within earshot. If a frightening word such as "cancer" is used in the medical discussion, patients panic. Even if the physician is saying that there is no possibility of cancer, patients may focus on a single word or phrase and not realize the context in which it is being used. Don't let fear stand in your way—bedside discussions do offer an opportunity to get more information. You have every right to interrupt and address the attending physician:

"When you were talking about surgery, you said a lot of things that scared me and that I don't really understand. I heard you mention cancer. Were you talking about me?"

The Visitor

When you are in the hospital, your human link with real life on the outside is the visitor. Family and friends call on the telephone and come to visit. Talking to them is a lifeline. There is a world beyond the hospital. Telephone calls are also welcome, even though they may interrupt the one nap you've had all day. Remember, you do have the option of having the nurse in charge block your calls so that you can receive them at your own convenience.

As far as actual visits, there is good news and bad news. Obviously, it's wonderful to see the people you know and care about. But, as a patient, you are already obligated to the hospital staff who cares for you and who want to be appreciated, and then the visitors may also expect gratitude and appreciation. They sometimes arrive with fragrant flowers for which you don't have a vase, present you with candy you can't eat, and magazines you don't want to read. So, while patients do enjoy and need to see family and friends for emotional support, I have also observed patients not knowing how to deal with visitors or how to get out of visits politely.

From the point of view of the patient, flat in bed, there is little choice about who comes to visit, when, or for how long. Patients worry about the fact that they haven't been able to make themselves presentable. They often feel embarrassed, tired, trapped, and without control over the subject of conversation. Some visitors make unintentional tactless remarks:

"Aren't you lucky, all you have to do is lie here all day. You should only know what kind of a day I had!"

Others may ask insensitive questions about the illness:

"So, now that you've had a hysterectomy, is it true that you'll have to take hormone injections for the rest of your life?"

Or they may criticize the care you're receiving:

"Oh, they put you in a terrible little room! Couldn't you have gotten one with a bigger window? Gee, is that the bathroom they expect you to use?"

Again, these are issues that are out of the patient's control, but are apt to be taken personally. When visitors criticize the hospital or health care, the patient who is dependent on it and has no alternatives ends up feeling obliged to defend it.

The situation is not always a comfortable one from the visitor's point of view either. Visitors sometimes doubt whether they should even be there and feel out of place. They are acutely aware of all the pain and illness around them. Unlike the staff and even some of the more seasoned patients, they may be overwhelmed. And if, as a visitor, you see something that you believe is not good for the person you've come to see, you're in a bind. You'd like to complain, but are afraid it will reflect on the patient and cause them to get worse care. If you don't say anything, you worry whether everything will be all right. There is a strong temptation to get into the act. When patients say:

"I wanted to ask the doctor, but he was in such a hurry I didn't get to," visitors are prone to respond:

> *"Why didn't you ask that? You really should! Why don't you call him or ask him to come back? Or would you like me to speak to him?"*

That's the last thing patients want visitors to do. And visitors are left thinking,

> *"I was only trying to help . . . ."*

There are two extremes of how visitors respond to seeing a person they know sick in a hospital bed. Although well intended, both can be hard on the patient. One is to express a lot of pity:

> *"Oh, you poor thing, you can't move and you have to be flat on your back and it must be very painful . . . ,"*

which only makes the patient feel worse. The opposite extreme is to be callous and minimize the patient's discomfort and assume the patient can take it:

> *"Oh, you'll be fine! I'm not that worried about you. You're tough."*

Sometimes visitors inadvertently make the patient feel like a burden:

> *"I should have been here earlier, but I've been so busy."*

"I really was in pain—it seemed like forever. How can I let you know if I need you urgently?"

When you feel you need to go to a higher authority—and this you should save for special issues—speak to the nursing supervisor, but try not to venture out of the nursing system. For instance, if you were to speak to the superintendent of the hospital, things might only get worse. Try to put yourself in the nurse's position. Let's say she was really busy with a very sick patient in another room and wasn't able to come to your room. Then you complain to the superintendent who's sitting in a comfortable office and calls her in. How sympathetic will she be to your complaints after she has lost face? Before you use any power tactics, try to solve the problem by relating directly to the individuals involved, respecting their professional competence, and politely insisting that your concerns be dealt with. This gets trickier and trickier in larger hospitals where more personnel is involved. Very few of the professional staff members with whom you have contact will be there for you every day. In spite of that, try to know people's names and form relationships with them. Respect them as individuals and express your appreciation.

Use your communication skills to make an alliance with one of the nurses or one of the aids. Hospitalization becomes more tolerable if you can find one person with whom you have a special relationship and who then may act as your advocate. Even though it's the nurse's responsibility to take care of you, if he or she gives you any special service or is skillful in doing something for you, don't hesitate to express your appreciation. Just as in any other situation, people will make a greater effort if they perceive that they are being noticed and appreciated.

Taking Charge

On record there are a couple of glorious exceptions to the lack of control most people experience in the hospital. For instance, as he describes in his book *The Anatomy of an Illness,* Norman Cousins managed to virtually take over the hospital and staff who cared for him in his belief that laughing and humor could cure even serious illness.[1] He dictated what his doctors could and could not do, provided himself with humorous reading and Marx Brothers films in his room to keep himself laughing, and altogether created a hospital existence that suited his tastes and fit his own philosophy about health and disease.

Another patient, world-renowned nuclear physicist Leo Szilard, also managed to do things his own way at a distinguished New York hospital.[2] Instead of accepting the hospital's rules and style, he imposed his own personality on the setting. He ordered food brought in from some of the best restaurants in New York. He pulled the shades down so that doctors and staff could not look in on him the way they usually do in hospitals. He put up a "Do Not Disturb" sign when he did not wish to be interrupted; he prohibited blood drawing and other annoying procedures at the crack of dawn. And once he found out what his disease was, he recruited several hospital staff members to work part time as his research assistants and had them spending hours down in the medical library exploring the best treatment for his condition.

Cousins and Szilard were able to turn the dominating and alienating hospital world around to their advantage. Although most of us do not have their resources or prestige, let us not forget their examples. There are always options to explore and decisions to make on our own. It's important to be a good observer, watch for opportunities, and reach out to those who are providing care. But it is not necessarily the arrogant, complaining, aggressive patients who get the best of care. Instead, the advantage goes to those who are sensitive enough to be able to put themselves in the position of the health-care professionals while at the same time articulately express feelings, opinions, and preferences.

There are, of course, many insults to privacy, independence, and comfort that are inevitable in any medical setting. But alternatives do exist and opportunities can be seized by the patient without offending caretakers. Remember that you don't catch bees with vinegar. You may not be able to order in take-out food, but you may be able to explain to the dietitian that you prefer vegetarian meals. If you've had a bad night, the next morning you can inquire whether for once some of the routine tests can be postponed. Although you may not be able to muster a team of research assistants to learn more about your condition, there are other options. Ask the doctor for more explanation and inquire as to whether there are magazine articles, books, or videos on the subject. You may not have the audacity to put a "Do Not Disturb" sign on the door, but if you want to visit with someone privately, you might ask the nurse or another staff member whether they could keep your door closed for a while. Negotiate quiet time with your roommate if you are bothered with the television programs he or she is watching. And inquire about the hospital's libraries—they often have good choices in books and movies on video. In many small ways, every patient has the option of making things more tolerable.

Outpatient Surgery

When one patient told her roommate that she was going to have breast surgery, her roommate asked, *"How long will you be in the hospital? How can I help?"* The patient told her that she had been stunned to learn that the procedure was going to be done on an outpatient basis:

"Can you imagine that? They tell me I'll be home the same day!"

More and more surgeries and other complex procedures are now being performed on an outpatient basis. Some of these you would never have dreamt could be done without a prolonged hospital stay.

Patients check in on the morning when surgery is scheduled and do not spend the night in the hospital. After the operation, they find themselves back at home, basically on their own, although nurses are sometimes scheduled for brief home visits to change dressings and manage medications and IVs. In this situation, patients need family or good friends for support, because they are on their own. And even if they are doing well, it is hard to take care of basic needs alone—such as going to the store for food and preparing meals.

What does this mean for you? Since having to be in the hospital is one of the most uncomfortable, disenfranchising, frightening things for all of us, outpatient surgery has many advantages. All other things being equal, of course it is nicer to be at home than in the hospital. We have also learned that limiting bed rest and making every effort to allow the patient to resume a normal life as soon as possible promotes recovery. And, in many ways, outpatient surgery has made the whole business of having an operation less dramatic.

Is that good? Yes and no. Going into the hospital, having an operation, and being hospitalized meant that you became part of a big ritual and a drama that somehow distanced you from the experience. You became a "real" patient and went through the experience as a patient. Now, as an outpatient, it's you as a person who goes through it all. In some ways, that makes it more threatening.

You present yourself at the hospital very early in the morning in your own clothes, upright and alert. Before, if you had been hospitalized prior to the surgery, you might have felt dehumanized and depersonalized, but somehow it didn't hit as close to home. When a patient is in the operating room, undressed, flat-out, draped, and anesthetized, it removes the personal element and allows the surgeon and staff to be more objective and professional. And, in a sense, that is true from the patient's side too. But when you arrive at the hospital on the morning of your surgery, march in, undress, and go through the surgery, it makes for a different mind-set. It is really *you* going through the experience, not someone who has had the time to adjust to being a "patient." You are more of a participant. But when you are hospitalized, from the moment you go in, you are sedated and taken care of and abandon yourself to the care of the hospital. Although some patients prefer outpatient surgery, for others it is much harder to complete the transition from being a person to being a patient and then suddenly back again.

Patients who were in the hospital for an operation in the old days also got quite a bit of mileage out of the fact that this was a dramatic event. Patients said bravely, "I'm going under the knife!" They got flowers, nurses to take care of them, visitors, and get-well cards. After surgery, they found themselves in a recovery room until they were wheeled back to their own room. Patients and family waited with suspense until the surgeon came to see them and told them how the operation went. Later, the daily visits from the surgeon with careful attention to the incision, general advice, and finally the welcome news that the patient was able to get out of bed and ultimately go home. And lots of interest from everyone as to "how many stitches?"—with numerous stitches being more prestigious than just a few.

What Is Outpatient Surgery Like?

Most of the drama is gone. Can you imagine yourself having a good night's sleep alone at home the night before the operation? One patient complained:

"I thought I was going to have a heart attack because my heart was pounding wildly all night! And I told my husband so. He, of course, thought I was crazy."

Admittedly, not too many patients have very restful nights before surgery in the hospital either, but for better or worse, they are usually sedated and help is available down the hall.

For day surgery, you are scheduled to present yourself at the crack of dawn. You get up reluctantly after an uneasy night, may not know what to wear, what to bring, what to anticipate. You may not be sure whether you will be able to drive "afterward," so you try to find someone who doesn't mind waiting for an uncertain period of time. Are you imposing? Somehow since you will be coming home the same day, it does not really seem justified to ask friends to inconvenience themselves.

There is no ceremony to mark this occasion, yet for you it is still an event filled with fear and uncertainty. Will it hurt? How will the anesthetic be given? How will you feel after it wears off and you're back home? Will you know what to watch for? Will you be able to eat? You probably were not allowed to eat anything since the night before, and right now you are too nervous to be hungry. But isn't it bad to have everything done on an empty stomach just when you need your strength? You wish you had eaten more the night before, but you just didn't have an appetite. Should you have had that glass of wine before dinner? Nobody said not to, but maybe they figured that you would know that it was not the thing to do.

Nevertheless, you set off for the hospital or the doctor's office where the deed will be done. Riding through empty streets, you observe other people beginning their daily routines and wish you were one of them. Anyone but you. Then when you arrive, your first duty is to sign a million papers and forms, mostly about your insurance policy, but also some that tell you that the hospital or medical center not only does not take any responsibility for your possessions, but also declines liability for all kinds of medical mishaps that could occur. You have questions you would like to ask, but soon it becomes apparent that most of the people who might have the answers have not yet arrived on the scene. Why did you bother to get there so early?

You ask when your friend can come and pick you up, but no one knows. They just say that he should call later in the day to find out. Call where? When? Then you are taken into another area and told to take off all your clothes. Undress? How far? All the way—for eye surgery? While you sit on the edge of the bed with nothing to do, not even a magazine to look at, all you can do is ask yourself whether you really need to be there . . . maybe you should have gotten another opinion?

In slow procession, other people come in to do things to you. Temperature, blood pressure (it must be sky high by this point!), blood tests, and so it goes. It seems like hours—and you could have stayed at home in bed.

The time seems to drag at first and then, all of a sudden, things start to happen very fast. They take on a momentum of their own. You think, *I'm not really ready for this,* but there is no further negotiation. You may be given a sedative immediately and not know what happens after that. Or, an attendant appears and quickly pushes you down a lot of corridors, into an elevator or two where other hospital staff look down at you, then off you go speeding down more corridors and through more swinging doors until you reach the operating suite. When you enter that chilly atmosphere with its tiled walls and empty corridors, you may be kept flat on your back for a while. Busy people rush by, calling out jocular greetings to one another or exchanging technical details:

> *"I guess he'll have to wait here, the doc in there is having some unexpected problems."*

Now there is no escape—you're next!

Once you are wheeled into the actual operating room, at least you feel that everybody there is getting ready to pay attention to you. The staff will probably introduce themselves and even tell you what they are about to do. Someone may give you a warm blanket if you ask for it.

Whenever possible, physicians choose to use local rather than general anesthesia because it's safer for the patient and avoids unpleasant after effects. On the other hand, it introduces a new set of problems because the patient is awake during the procedure and hears the surgeons and nurses comment on what they're doing. The comments are often in technical language and can be alarming:

> *"Don't you think you need to go into the next intervertebral space?"*
> *"I think you're going too high . . . ."*
> *"Let me have the suction. I need it <u>now</u>."*
> *"What are you looking for?"*

Even though the local anesthetic usually controls actual pain, you are still aware of what is being done. You may be uncomfortable and feel pressure and manipulation. You may also be in a very awkward position. Often patients have to be immobilized; sandbags may be placed on your body or around your head for procedures that require you to be absolutely motionless. Although it's not painful, it can be alarming to be restrained for a long period of time. A patient told me:

> "One of the things I find the most scary about local anesthesia is that you're afraid you might do something that will keep them from being able to do as well as they might. I remember how they said don't move, don't breathe . . . and then I was scared to death. I was immobilized in every way and it was my eye . . . I was afraid if I moved at all, if I flinched, that I might cause a problem."

In a sense you are still a participant, but you have to accept that you are in competent hands. There is no point in trying to second guess because it will probably only make things worse. Remind yourself that you are there to get help with a problem and that everyone there is doing their best and wishing you well. There are times to question and assert yourself, and there are times to accept and try to relax. This is definitely one where you need to relax and put your trust in your doctor.

Being Prepared for Outpatient Surgery

From the moment when the operation is first mentioned by your doctor, you must get into an inquiring mode. Don't be afraid of being thought ignorant. Why should you have known about the particular procedure until you were actually faced with it? When you go to see the doctor for the last time before the surgery, take full advantage of that visit. Inquire about what is involved and find out who else you can ask. Many patients find it helpful to talk to someone else who has had a similar experience. Remember that information from other patients, although it can be helpful, can also be misleading. Procedures can be different and the response of one patient does not necessarily predict how you will feel. Still, if you want to get another patient's point of view, that's the way to go. It has been said that the difference between major and minor surgery is that when it's you, it's major.

Remember that you, the patient, are a part of the decision-making process. Feel free to ask relevant questions:

"Why am I having outpatient surgery instead of being admitted into the hospital?"
"Is it for financial reasons?"
"What are the risks?"
"What are the benefits?"
"Is there an urgency?"
"How much time will it take?"

You should make your decisions in full awareness of all the implications for you as a patient. If, in the face of what you are told, your choice is not to go, that is an option.

If possible, ask the doctor about the hospital's consent forms ahead of time so you don't have surprises at the last minute. Although your physician may not have the official forms, he or she will probably have a general idea of what's going to be asked. If you would like to go over the actual forms ahead of time, the doctor's office may be able to help you obtain copies if you ask far enough in advance.

When you arrive at the hospital, if you are confronted with papers to sign at the last minute—slid across the table by someone who probably does not know much more than you do about the actual medical procedure—again do not hesitate to ask questions. If there is something you do not understand, make sure you insist on talking with someone who does know before you sign anything. While it may not make you popular, any responsible person should welcome your wanting to make an informed decision rather than being blindly compliant.

When it comes to being sedated or even anesthetized, you need to find out what drugs are being used and what you can expect. If you have concerns, talk to your doctor during the last visit before you go in for the surgery. Then, when you are in the hospital, talk to the anesthesiologist. Even if you did talk to the doctor beforehand, the staff may be unaware that you are unusually sensitive or even allergic to a particular drug. In any case, you should ask questions so that you understand the purpose of the drug that will be used. Is the goal to keep you sound asleep during the procedure or will you just be drowsy? Are you expected to feel anything at all? Pain?

Pressure? Should you speak up if you do? Basically, you have a right to be kept from having any real pain, unless you are a stoic type who prefers to be as aware as possible and would rather tolerate pain and discomfort than being heavily sedated.

One patient, Amy, was recently scheduled for eye surgery and the doctor automatically assumed that she would want the usual sedation. She took advantage of the available opportunities and managed to get the necessary information. The doctor even respected her preferences concerning the routine procedure for sedation:

> "I asked him [the doctor] about radial keratotomy, which I had been considering. He discussed it quite thoroughly. His assistant then gave me more information and set up an appointment for the pre-op visit. Most of the exam was done by an assistant who seemed capable.
>
> "I was shown a video about the RK and the assistant answered questions. Actually, the video did make me a little apprehensive because it showed the patient in a hospital gown and looking rather woozy.
>
> "The office was supposed to send information about the RK a week before my appointment, but I did not receive it. So I called the office and the assistant went over the information with me over the phone. One thing that I had not been aware of was that I would be given Valium before the RK and sleeping pills for that night. I told her that I had had unpleasant experiences with sedatives and would rather have the surgery without any. She talked to the doctor, came back to the phone, and said he was willing to do the RK without sedatives.
>
> "Surgery was interesting . . . I was given anesthetic eye drops and experienced no pain at all. When I went in the next morning for a checkup, the doctor said my vision was already 20/30, better than he had expected. He asked if I had been apprehensive about not being sedated and I said not at all . . . . Then he told me that he had been pretty nervous about it!"

After Your Surgery

Another critical time is when you wake up after the procedure and want to know how it went and what they found. By the time you really wake up, it seems as if everyone but you has left the premises. No one who was actually present at the procedure is available to talk to you. You ask the nurse,

"How did it go?"

she says,

"Everything went fine, you have nothing to worry about."

You ask,

"Were you there?"

and find out that she wasn't, but that her reports and the chart indicate everything went routinely. Routinely? When it's your body, it is never routine. You want to hear what they did, what they found—and you want to hear it from someone who was actually there and knows.

At that point in the day, it may be hard for the staff in the recovery room to actually get ahold of your doctor. If you had enough forethought, you could have made arrangements during your last office visit for a telephone call after surgery. If the operation took place early enough, you may be able to speak with her that same day while she's still at the hospital or back in her office. But if the procedure took place later in the day or you had heavy sedation, request that the doctor call you when you get home.

For a while after the procedure, you will probably be drowsy and drift in and out of sleep. And then suddenly you are told that your friend is there to pick you up. You may not feel prepared to leave yet. One patient commented,

"I did not feel mentally ready, I felt really shaky on my feet, it seemed like days since I put my clothes on that morning. I felt like I was returning from another world."

There is a tendency for people not to take outpatient surgery seriously:

"Oh, I guess your operation isn't very serious if it's only day surgery."

Yet for you, it's a tremendous experience. One patient told me,

> *"Doctors don't realize that even if someone just sticks a needle in your finger, for you that's serious!"*

And having someone operate on you, whether on an outpatient basis or during a prolonged hospital stay, is serious no matter how you look at it.

While it's probably better for the patient not to be in the hospital overnight, and most patients are glad not to have to stay, on the other hand, don't fool yourself. Outpatient surgery is still a big assault on your body and your identity. In some ways it is especially disorienting because the ritual is gone. One moment you are being taken into an operating room, the next you find yourself back in a car and on the street. The key to getting through the experience is preparing ahead of time and then relaxing. It pays to be a well-informed, self-assertive patient. Before you schedule daytime surgery, it's up to you to take care of yourself. So be sure to talk to the doctor about the anesthesia, the consent forms, the arrangements, and remember that your initial relief—

> *"Oh good, I'm not going to have to stay in the hospital."*

has to be tempered with,

> *"What do I need to do to prepare myself?"*

Here is a short checklist to keep in mind if outpatient surgery is in your future:

- ▾ Bring a friend, or have someone pick you up. You shouldn't drive yourself home or have to take public transportation when you will probably still not be yourself.

- ▾ Wear clothes that you can get in and out of easily. If you're having eye surgery, for example, don't wear a tight pullover sweater. If you are having an abdominal incision, don't wear something with a tight waist. If it's your knee that's going to be operated on, wear loose pants or gym shorts.

▼ Stock your refrigerator and have meals on hand that are easy to prepare and heat up.

▼ If your living quarters are on more than one floor, make arrangements so that you don't have to climb the stairs.

▼ Ask your doctor what to expect: How often do you need to take medication? When should you change your bandages? Are there any other instructions? If your doctor is not available, find out who can answer your questions. In most instances, there will be written instructions available at the hospital or clinic where you will have the surgery; if not, make sure that everything is written down. At home, you may not be able to remember.

▼ Are there other people at home who depend on you? Children? Pets? Be sure to make arrangements so that their needs (and yours!) will be taken care of.

▼ Depending on the seriousness of the procedure, you may decide that making all these arrangements is too much for you. If so, find someone else to do it for you.

▼ Make sure you know how to reach the doctor and his or her personnel after you get home.

GETTING THE MOST OUT
OF MANAGED CARE

▼
▼

*Three doctors wait at the Pearly Gates, all in hopes of gaining
entry. St. Peter asks the first one, a private practitioner, "What
have you done to deserve admittance to these hallowed grounds?"
He replies, "I have treated the ill, I have relieved their pain and
saved many lives." St. Peter responds enthusiastically, "You have
done well, my child, come on in!" When asked the same question,
the next doctor responds, "I have been working in public health
clinics all my life and cared for needy patients." Hearing this,
St. Peter approves and welcomes him through the gate with, "Oh
yes, you also have done much good, my child, come in." When the
third doctor pleads his case, "I too have devoted my life to caring for
the sick. I have helped many, many patients in the years that I have
worked as a staff member at an HMO." St. Peter smiles, opens the
gates, and responds, "You may come in but your stay will be limited to three days."*

St. Peter blames the doctor for the new rules and restrictions imposed by
managed health care—as many of us do. But is that really fair? He deserves
to go to heaven too; he has worked hard and probably made less money than
most physicians in private practice. What this story does reflect are our con-

cerns about the way in which HMOs make decisions. Managed care is planned for large populations, not individuals. And a common complaint about HMOs is that you are dismissed from the hospital before you are ready.

Your stay will be determined depending on your diagnosis and what needs to be done. You may be entitled to five days, perhaps only three, or the decision may be that your problem can be handled on an outpatient basis. Unfortunately, no one has devoted sufficient attention to how you will respond as an individual. Being sent home twenty-four hours after surgery is scary. There is very little leeway in terms of individual needs. Women who have given birth have been booted out of many hospitals after only eighteen hours. Without a chance to recover from the delivery, they may be overwhelmed, tired, not ready to care for the baby without help. What's more, if anything goes wrong with the baby in the first week, no professional is there to observe it. Previously, problems like newborn jaundice were usually picked up during the time the baby was in the hospital.

The following is an excerpt from an interview with a mother whose infant had numerous severe medical problems. Her baby was kept in the newborn intensive-care unit for many weeks. She was not prepared when she suddenly found out that her baby was ready to go home:

> *"It was very startling. You work toward this goal of getting home, it's all you think of . . . . And the first time someone said it [that we were going home] to me, I said—"Are you kidding?" I didn't want any part of it . . . I thought, 'There's no way I can do this!'*
>
> *"They set a release date for him and I hadn't finished learning all the procedures. I went through a reverse thing where I felt rejected. And purely by coincidence, I'm sure, our insurance was running out. I felt, fine, our insurance is going good-bye, out the door. And I hadn't even learned what I was doing yet. I got very scared at the end.*
>
> *"Our child had been watched virtually every minute of every day, whether it had been by machine or by actual nurses being there. And suddenly I was going to take him home, and I didn't feel comfortable with everything that I had been taught. We were there with a list of emergencies the day we were having the party for him to go home. So there was no time to even go over them, think about them, come back with questions.*

"I sort of felt like I was shoved out the door. At the end, I wanted out the door desperately, but it was just rough."

In the past, patients were often kept in the hospital too long. It's a lot easier, for instance, for a doctor to see a series of patients between 7:30 and 8:00 A.M. and send them each a bill than to schedule them all separately in the office. And you may not realize that for a hospital, in view of all the services that have to be available at all times, there is nothing more expensive than keeping an empty bed. But that reason for hospitalization is no longer acceptable under managed care.

Our health-care system is in flux. Some things are reasonable, others are not. Since hospitalization isn't pleasant and is extremely costly, in many cases, shorter stays may be a good thing. Unfortunately, adequate provisions are often not made for the much needed support of patient and family following early discharge. You may suddenly learn that it is time to go home, but there have been no arrangements made for getting there. You are unable to drive, have not had the opportunity to call someone to pick you up, are told it's time to go, and find yourself stuck. Or perhaps something has happened at home that makes going there difficult. A mother, for instance, is about to be discharged with her newborn baby and finds out that one of her children at home has just developed chicken pox. Even though chicken pox is not a life-threatening disease, it might be risky for the new baby to be exposed.

We're in the process of change and it's not always clear what can be changed and what you have to accept. Within a very short time, two patients talked to me about their hospital experience. One told about begging to stay an extra day after a mastectomy and not being given the opportunity. Another patient told me that she simply mentioned that she felt a little weak after childbirth, asked for an extra day, and her HMO doctor arranged it. If a patient is discharged prematurely and suffers from a serious complication, then the health-care plan *and* the individual doctor are held accountable. Not long ago a patient was hospitalized for a surgical procedure and was abruptly discharged two days later. The following day, he developed a serious complication and died. His family successfully sued not only the health-care plan but also the physician who had not intervened to keep him in the hospital. Remember, your doctor can serve as your advocate in the health-care system.

Roadblocks

> *"When I used to go see my regular doctor, it certainly was more convenient. Now what I have to go through to get there makes me wonder whether I'll even be willing to go."*

The experience of visiting the doctor's office certainly is undergoing some brutal changes. An elderly patient, Mr. L., who has cancer, has gone to the same physician for decades, but recently was forced to endure some changes:

> *"My doctor's office was in a small, two-story medical building close to where I live. It was on the ground floor, not very large or elegant, but I felt comfortable there. I knew both the doctor and the nurse well, and if I needed to talk to them about anything, I could call anytime. But when my doctor had to join an HMO, he moved to one of those big buildings.*
>
> *"You have to park underground and it's very confusing. There are so many elevators going to different parts of the building that every time I go I have a hard time figuring out which one I'm supposed to take. Even the nurse who works with Dr. H. complains to me that she feels alienated. She told me the other day that she was thinking of quitting."*

The patient was getting more and more debilitated and found the changes so disturbing that he wasn't sure whether he would be able to continue his long-standing relationship with his doctor:

> *"I'm a very independent person. I've always taken care of myself. With the office so far away and inconvenient, it's almost impossible for me to get there. I used to just walk into town on the way to his office and on the way home stop at the grocery to get some essentials. It took me a half hour each way.*
>
> *"Now, he's so far away that if I try to walk over there, as sick as I am, it takes me almost two hours. I have to walk on a very busy, high traffic road, and I'm exhausted when I get there. Since I am no longer able to drive myself . . . I either have to ask for a ride or walk and so I've resigned myself . . . I have to beg for rides."*

The physical layout of HMO offices is often perceived by patients as unfriendly. What has been lost is the individualized feeling. Patients are corralled into place to contend with inhospitable barriers: large sterile counters, glass partitions, closed doors, white corridors, and mazes. The pictures on the walls may not be your doctor's choice. Previously, you might have liked your doctor's taste in art; you might have thought, *Oh, she likes impressionists too.* Now, large offices are decorated by design firms and don't represent the tastes of either patient or doctor. One patient commented,

> *"In my doctor's new office, they have this extravagant, large aquarium with exotic fish and fancy lights that cover an entire wall. I miss the familiar round glass bowl with its two little goldfish."*

Despite this new atmosphere, these large medical office suites have some advantages. Many more things are easily accessible. Specialists may be right down the hall instead of miles away in another office. Lab tests can be done more efficiently at no extra inconvenience to you. Technical services such as X ray or EKG are likely to be readily available. That means you don't have to drive across town and wrestle with all the inconveniences of another medical plaza. You now have one-stop-shopping service!

Why Can't I Choose My Own Doctor?

> *"I feel trapped in my health plan. I have to limit myself to their doctors, their specialists, and their tests. I can't go anywhere else."*

While there is justification for this complaint, the reality is that there are positives and negatives. We hear a lot nowadays about the good old days before managed health care when everything was so lovely. Well, it wasn't all lovely. The ideal one-to-one relationship between patient and doctor in the past was the exception rather than the rule. There are age-old problems relating to the complex relationships between patient and physician. It is, of course, a myth that most patients always got tender, loving, individualized care. Before managed care, many people did not even have a doctor or a particular institution that they related to. When asked,

> *"Do you ever go in for a checkup?"*

they stopped and thought and finally said,

"No."

When something went wrong, they had to scout around, ask their friends for recommendations, or sometimes went to a specialist they knew, which was inappropriate.

Not many people have anything nice to say about HMOs—*"HMOs make me sick! You can't even choose your own doctor!"*—but, at present, most people are able to identify who their primary care physician is or at least the medical care system to which they belong.

Previously patients believed that, with an unlimited choice of physicians, they would end up with the best one. Now they fear that they will have to settle for less. But in the past people often used inappropriate criteria in choosing their physicians—they looked in the Yellow Pages or perhaps sought out friends and co-workers for recommendations. Recently a patient told her physician that he had been recommended by the person waiting behind her in line at the supermarket. In light of that, the current situation is not necessarily bad. Many managed health-care organizations evaluate their physicians carefully before they employ them and monitor the quality of care they give. So you are guaranteed a level of confidence that you couldn't count on before.

Remember that nothing you actually had before has really been cut out. If you are not satisfied with the answers your doctors are giving, you have a right to a second opinion and there is also the option of going to a physician outside the system. If, for example, you are having a symptom and feel strongly that you need to see a specialist or have certain tests and your HMO refuses, then you can still make an appointment for a consultation with a private practitioner if you are willing to pay for it. If it does turn out that you do, in fact, need to undergo treatment or surgery, it may be available through your original plan.

Elective surgeries are a different matter. Managed health-care organizations prioritize on the basis of medical necessities. If you can afford it, you can, of course, have anything you want. If, for instance, you've never liked the shape of your nose and now you want to fix it, your HMO will most probably not do it. And they probably also won't be very open to providing you with the latest shade of tinted contact lenses. But you still can go to the nearest plastic surgeon or optometrist, have the procedure done, and pay for it on your own just as you used to.

Where do HMO doctors come from? Do you ever stop to think that the doctors who work in HMOs are the same "private" physicians that all of us have been seeing for years? There are, at present, very few doctors who are able to maintain a strictly private practice. There is no new species being bred to work at HMOs! Except that now they have to go through new screening processes and periodic reviews. Private physicians were never dismissed for failure to practice optimal medicine. HMO physicians do run that risk because their performance is closely scrutinized. Patients have a great fear that physicians in managed care organizations will be predictably less personal and less individualizing. But do you think that physicians who are properly trained and have the right values are really going to change their basic attitudes toward patients just because they are working at HMOs? They may be angry and frustrated at the system, but don't forget that years ago physicians might have been angry because the rent was being raised on their medical suites, malpractice premiums were increasing, or scheduling difficulties were becoming unmanageable.

Be careful that you, the patient, don't change your own attitude toward a physician just because he or she works in an HMO. If you approach your new doctor with the same respect that you extended to your private physician, he or she will be more likely to go out of the way for you. Because physicians are no longer specifically chosen by patients, they feel less special. While you may feel offended because the plan made the assignment for you, the physician may also feel less valued. Unfortunately, patients are now less likely to express their individual appreciation for the services they receive because they feel entitled to these services, and, when their expectations aren't met, they feel shortchanged and take it out on the physician. If you have been especially well taken care of, it is appropriate to let the physician know or even to tell the organization so that he or she gets the feedback.

Will I Ever See the Same Physician Twice?

Yes, you can request the doctor you wish to see when you call for an appointment, and, if you can wait, you usually will succeed. Many of us overlook the fact that, even before, there were occasions when our doctors were not on call. But in a well-running HMO, the physicians are long-term employees and, in most instances, you will be able to see the same doctor. Continuity of care has consistently been shown to improve patient follow-through. We all know it's easier to talk to a physician you know than someone you've never seen before, especially when it comes to sensitive subjects. When enrolling into a new system, it is essential to foster a relationship with an individual physician and, in some cases, it may be equally important to know the main nurse practitioner or associate health professional with whom he or she works. The system can't legislate a relationship—it's up to you. You'd be surprised how many people call up and don't even know the name of their doctor. There's nothing to keep you from saying,

"May I have your name and your card please?"

Be sure that you are able to ask for both the doctor and nurse by name.

It takes time to develop enough trust in a physician to be comfortable. It also takes time for the physician to know you: what to expect from you, what is acceptable to you and what is not, how to elicit information from you most effectively, and so on.

An acquaintance mentioned that her doctor had given her a new medication and that she was confused about some new symptoms. She told me:

"I don't know whether I'm feeling this way from the side effects of the medication or whether I'm having new symptoms."

I replied,

"Well, you should discuss that with your doctor."

Her response:

"I can't do that. I'm HMO."

The implication was that there was a gigantic barrier keeping her from speaking to her doctor. It does take some work for patients to learn the system, to know their doctors well enough to feel comfortable, and to know how to reach their doctors—but it can be done.

in the medical visit than how much time the doctor actually spent. This is why it is so important for patient and physician to develop good communication skills. In one of our studies, we measured the time physicians actually spent in the examination room with patients and compared it with how much time patients thought the doctor had spent.[1] Even after long visits, patients who were dissatisfied complained that the doctor had seemed in a hurry. But when things went well and patients were satisfied, they tended to overestimate the time the doctor had actually devoted.

Why Can't I See a Specialist?

One of the complaints heard most frequently from HMO patients is that they are not able to go directly to the specialist of their choice:

> "I wanted to see my gynecologist the way I used to but I found out I couldn't make the appointment with him, I had to see someone else first."

Patients resent not being able to go directly to a specialist. In traditional medical practice, if you wanted to see an orthopedist or a gynecologist, you simply made an appointment. Managed care practice, on the other hand, is structured on the basis of policies developed for a population of patients.

Having to accept the decision of the primary-care physician as to whether you can see a specialist may make you feel as if you've lost control. But when you think about it, going directly to a specialist for a specific complaint implies that you as the patient are always able to diagnose the exact nature of your problem. Although you may feel you can do that, surprisingly often specialists see patients with symptoms that are not in their area of expertise and that could have been better and more easily diagnosed and treated by a general physician.

If you have a rash, for instance, and are certain that you need to see a dermatologist, you may actually be wrong. Not every rash is just a skin problem; it may be a manifestation of a generalized disease. To take an obvious example, measles is due to a generalized infection, not a skin problem. And while one of the symptoms of lupus is a rash, a dermatologist would not be the best physician to see because it is a serious disease internists are best trained to manage. In fact, most of the things that are simple enough to diagnose yourself can be taken care of perfectly well by a primary-care doctor. If all you need are cool soaks of permanganate on your blisters or hydrocortisone ointment on an itchy rash, you really don't require a dermatologist.

I recently saw a child who went to a major department store to have glasses prescribed. The optometrist at the store noticed something unusual with her eyes and sent her to an ophthalmologist. The ophthalmologist recognized that this was not an eye problem, but part of a generalized condition and sent her to a pediatrician. This was indeed backwards—from the glasses counter to the specialist to the generalist!

Physicians cannot always make referrals when they would like to. They have to operate within the rules of the system. There has been heated controversy over the "gag" rule that discouraged physicians in some HMOs from even discussing options with patients. However, it is your right to at least be informed of all the options, even if the particular health maintenance organization may not be able to provide all the services. Therefore, if you have a major complaint and feel strongly that you need to see a specialist, it's time to speak up. If you are denied a particular consultation, you as a patient have the right to be informed of all the options within the system and elsewhere. Remember, it is not only important for you but, logically, it is also in the best interest of the managed-care organization to make sure you get appropriate care. If you develop a serious medical condition with complications, it will not only be costly medically for the HMO, but also legally.

The system doesn't work for every patient. In this next interview, Mrs. X., the mother of a chronically ill child who is enrolled in a health-care maintenance organization, talks about the problems she has had. I've known her child, Linda, and her family ever since she was discharged from our newborn intensive-care unit after a seven-month hospitalization. She is dependent on a ventilator and for many years has needed a tracheotomy tube to enable her to breathe. Frustrated and discouraged, Mrs. X. is a well-educated "patient" who, with her husband, has consistently cared for their daughter twenty-four hours a day with the help of nurses and doctors. When she recognized that Linda had the symptoms of pneumonia, she called the doctor's office. She was not permitted to talk to a doctor directly and was unable to reach anyone who understood her child's condition. She was instructed to go to her managed-care clinic where everyone is seen first by triage nurses. She told me:

> *"When I call for extra help when Linda is ill, I'm usually denied that. I'm denied that and in addition I'm required to bring her in. I can understand that they want to see her, but when you bring in a child who is dependent on the ventilator—you should see us. We have a little red wagon that we put in the trunk, I take the red wagon out when we get to the clinic, I put Linda's blanket down and I put a ventilator in there, I put Linda in front of it, and now that she is six, we're just about full. But on top of that, I add my suction machine and I add a pulmo-aid for giving aerosol treatments, because it always involves a long wait."*

Although Mrs. X. knew more than most professionals about her child's condition, she was put through many unnecessary and inconvenient steps while her child was getting worse:

> *"One time about a year ago when I went in, I had to see the triage nurse first. I sat down opposite him and had Linda on my lap with her ventilator. The nurse leaned over, pointed to her tracheotomy, and asked, 'What is that little thing on her neck?' And I thought, 'This is the nurse that's triaging her to find out if she needs help! And he doesn't know a "trach" when he sees it!' And that's frightening. I just wish that they would believe me more as a mom, that when I call in and I say, 'This is happening, her lungs don't sound good, she's blue, I would like her to be seen by someone . . .' that they would believe me. I wish that I had a real doctor."*

Sometimes when I talked to Mrs. X. it seemed that she was almost suffering more from the pressures and inadequacies of the system than from the actual problems involved in her child's illness. During one particularly difficult period, she was so overwhelmed that she actually contemplated suicide. Looking back on that episode, one of her reactions was,

> *"Look what they've done to me . . . . Now what am I going to do?"*

Tests and Diagnostic Procedures

"Why can't I have a chest X ray? I've been coughing for three weeks after this flu!"

Patients feel cheated when doctors limit the number of tests and diagnostic procedures they can receive. This patient's HMO doctor did not order a chest X ray because, on examination, nothing indicated that it was necessary. A good primary physician knows that many patients cough for two to three weeks after the flu and so it would be a poor investment in time and money, and exposure to X rays is not entirely harmless. In the past, one of the most consistent patient complaints was that doctors were too quick to refer patients for tests, X rays, and consultations with other specialists. It was the individual physicians who made these decisions. They determined their patients' needs and sold their services accordingly:

"Come see me every week because I need to check your bloodwork."

In recent years, as physicians became more entrepreneurial and had additional services they could sell, things really got out of hand. There was no ceiling to how much they could charge patients, and they could invest in subsidiary technological activities such as X-ray labs and private hospitals that were financially rewarding. And you can imagine that if a doctor purchased his or her own expensive MRI equipment, it would have to be used in order to be paid for.

Even in recommending consultations, there was a possibility for self-serving interests. When referring patients to specialists, honest physicians would profit because it was good for the patient and it made for good relationships with the consultant who might return the referral. But there were even a few who split fees or got kickbacks.

"I heard that HMO doctors get bonuses for doing less for their patients."

Today as in the past, most physicians who choose to study medicine and practice it do so to help their patients. But the current climate in which diagnosis and treatment are sometimes a matter of policy rather than individual judgment have put the physician in a tremendous dilemma. In some organizations, physicians are limited in the number of consultations that can be recommended. In fact, they have limited budgets, which is where the term "gatekeeper" comes from. The "gates" are to be kept closed except when it's absolutely necessary to open them because the doctor is on a fixed budget. Overspending on consultations or tests can put a doctor at a financial disadvantage. There may be special incentives for doctors to stay within a budget, but if a doctor is negligent and something goes wrong, then that doctor is risking his or her career. Doctors consequently have less individual power because they are being told what to do. And if a patient requests something different, the doctor is in a bind. The HMO says, *"Don't do that!"* The patient says, *"Aren't you going to do it?"*

Both patients and practitioners have come to expect a whole array of technological tests as part of the doctor–patient encounter. This is one reason why health care became so expensive and that other systems are now evolving. So we are currently caught in a dilemma. Before we felt like victims when the doctor ordered a lot of tests, which left us wondering,

Do I really need all this? Why is he doing this?

And now we wonder,

Do I need tests and she's not ordering them just because I'm a patient in a managed-care plan?

In either case, patients are not sure what to believe.

What's in It for Me?

"It seems like I've lost a lot with the advent of managed care. The idea is to save money, but will it really cost me less?"

Yes, you probably will be spending less. It may be your employer who pays for part or all of your health-care plan or you may have a "co-pay" arrangement that means you pay a minimal fee for each visit and a small sum for prescriptions. In some organizations, the only change will be that you pay a lower price for each individual service as long as you operate within the system.

Among all the other confusions is the complex terminology that changes day to day—HMOs (Health Maintenance Organizations), IPAs (Independent Practice Associations), PPAs (Professional Practice Associations), MCOs (Managed Care Organizations), EPOs (Exclusive Provider Organizations), PPOs (Preferred Provider Organizations), and MSOs (Managed Service Organizations). Inform yourself before you join such an organization and know what the name stands for and what the ground rules are. Some are for-profit organizations that strive to make a profit for shareholders; others are nonprofit corporations for which the income goes back into patient care. One is not necessarily better than the other.

Managed-care plans may be based on capitation, which means that there is a set annual fee for each patient who is enrolled in the plan whether that patient is perfectly healthy or needs extensive care. Capitation is one of the forces that makes health-care plans competitive and eager to please these patients, because the more enrollees they have, the more money they make. If they have a great many members, they can afford to pay for expensive treatments for those who need them. If they are a smaller organization with fewer enrollees, some major mishaps like extensive surgeries and long hospitalizations can prove very costly. Thus, the bigness of the organization that patients so often complain about also carries benefits in terms of services available.

Just as we need to understand the laws of the community to which we belong, we all need to learn more about the constantly changing systems to which medical practice is subject. It becomes more and more important to explore our options for treatment, drugs, hospital care, outpatient care, home care, ambulatory therapy, specialist consultation, nurses in the home, and many others. There is a stream of information about all these subjects in the media, advertisements, books, and brochures. Every contract that you as a patient sign specifies limitations, exceptions, and benefits. It is often difficult to find your way through this maze of information and misinformation.

In general, it is wisest to stick with information generated within the practice to which you belong. Patients must be given a "patient's bill of rights," and there is a law that requires that patients be asked about "advance directives," which specify how they wish to handle critical events in their care.

Unfortunately, the language is often hard to understand. You must insist that you get interpretations. Do not be afraid to ask. You are not only entitled to understand, it is your responsibility to *yourself* to absolutely understand. If you are not satisfied with the information you have been given, find patient advocates and consult your doctor. Even your doctor may not have the answers you are looking for, but he or she can help you navigate. If you are told something that you find unacceptable—for instance, if you are not willing to have a particular procedure done as an outpatient with only local anesthesia—refuse and insist on finding out what the alternatives are. There is rarely only one way.

Paradoxically, new developments in health-care delivery reflect the need for cost effectiveness, while new developments in science and medical care go in the opposite direction. With all the breakthroughs, we have a tremendous amount of new knowledge: genetics and molecular biology, new chemotherapeutic agents, new antibiotics, new transplantation and surgical techniques, new technology for life support. Unfortunately, when this knowledge is applied to patient care, it rarely results in complete recovery, although it often prolongs life. The survivors of many of these drastic therapies live at great risk and may require extensive continuing care that adds astronomically to health-care costs. AIDS patients are living longer, but are tremendously vulnerable. People who have had transplants may have to be under close supervision for the rest of their lives. Cancer patients must endure radical surgery or treatment with fierce drugs that create complications. So there is a conflict: an explosion of new knowledge, whose application is very expensive, in the setting of an economically driven health-care system. Of all the new options for treatment, which ones are the insurers willing to pay for, and which ones won't they? How do we choose the right plan? Are you willing to pay twice the premium in case you need a kidney transplant? It is a distant possibility. Are you going to play the probabilities?

> *"I probably won't get that disease."*
> *"Why should I pay so much for the rest of my life for someone else to have a transplant?"*

It is up to you, but make sure you are informed in your choices.

Why Managed Care Needs to Keep Us Healthy

Even though this cost-conscious system might come across negatively in some of your own experiences as a patient, there are some good trends. One of the main benefits is the increasing emphasis on preventive medicine and health maintenance. For many, many years we complained that doctors weren't interested in keeping us healthy—they were just interested in treating disease.

We were the ones who had to take the initiative for keeping ourselves healthy and well—eating nutritious food, exercising, avoiding fat in our diets, you name it. But now, health care has switched gears and doctors have taken on the role of advocating wellness care partly out of humanism, but also because it reduces medical expenditures relating to medical visits, the number of times patients have to go to the hospital, the incidence of certain illnesses, and all the other things that make medical care so expensive. So it's the system and the doctors who have to be cost-conscious. In those organizations that are "capitated," a patient who stays well brings in the same amount of income per year as a patient who utilizes a lot of expensive health care, so there is a great advantage for the organization in having patients stay well. HMOs are initiating programs for preventive and screening measures such as immunizations and mammography, as well as patient education programs, all of which will reduce the incidence of illness as well as reduce the cost of caring for the patient over time.

Nowadays, hospitalization is being limited and much more is being done on an ambulatory basis. It's far less expensive for patients to make a short visit to the hospital for chemotherapy than live there for months, or for nurses and health professionals to make daily house calls for in-home IV treatments than for the hospital to provide full-time "hotel" service. From our point of view, these are improvements for patients. In pediatrics, certain hospitals have even organized "care-by-parent" wards where children are cared for in many ways by their parents instead of by paid professionals. These units are always provided with ready access to medical personnel, but bed-making, laundry, and meal service is done by parents. This makes the experience less frightening for the child and costs the hospital far less. Stressing prevention, lifestyle changes, and all the practices that keep people healthy is the very thing we, as patients, have been striving toward; it is also cost effective.

More and more, we need to turn our thinking around to look at the opportunities managed care will present instead of complaining. The changes were planned to meet a lot of unmet needs. Large groups in our community had no regular medical care whatsoever. With people being kept alive by life-support services, one-pound premature babies now surviving because of high-tech support systems, not to mention transplant and gene therapy, health care had become so astronomically expensive that very few individuals could afford to pay for it privately and it was a heavy burden on the community. Yet, those of us who have nothing but negative things to say about today's health care operate on the assumption that it could have gone on just the way it was forever. The reason it has changed is that it couldn't go on.

We are having new experiences that make us anxious but should ultimately bring about more attention to health and wellness than there was in the past. When medical practice was one-to-one, it tended to be disease and physician centered. Now, with different types of practices, there are some other important aspects of health care that are receiving more emphasis. One of these is the emphasis on keeping patients well and on preventive measures.

Another one is more focus on the doctor–patient relationship. Did you know that HMOs are monitoring physicians' communication skills, that there are courses in communication mandated for physicians in certain managed care organizations, and that patients are frequently given questionnaires about their physicians' performance and their own satisfaction? One of the main commodities health-care organizations have to sell is satisfaction, and if patients aren't happy—if we aren't happy—we won't like the plan and companies won't buy the plan.

Survival Tactics

Keep informed. Things are changing constantly, and there is no point sitting around and complaining. Managed care is a reality. You might as well complain about the fact that big cities are busy and have a lot of traffic. If you're a part of one, it's better to find out how to live with it and adapt than to complain.

One problem is that when we do have complaints and need help the most, we're usually sick and not in the frame of mind or position to do much about it. But when we get well and have distanced ourselves from the medical world, problems relating to our health care no longer seem so urgent. We have so many other things to deal with that seem to have higher priority. So, for your own sake and for the benefit of fellow sufferers, if you feel that there are areas needing intervention or correction, voice your concerns, even if it is after the fact. Nothing will change unless you speak up!

If you never want to see a particular doctor again, it is possible to find another doctor. But be careful about what you hold the doctor accountable for. If there are certain rules in the particular health plan, there's no use in wasting valuable time discussing it or even arguing with the doctor, because he or she is also operating in the same system and has to abide by the same rules you do. Instead, talk to the people who manage the plan. And talk to your employers if they are the ones who have subscribed to the plan. Look for opportunities to participate in decision making without causing open conflict. In all aspects of health care now, the system is accountable to the patient. If you have legitimate concerns, people will be interested in hearing what you have to say. If you become confused with too much conflicting information, ask for help.

Since we are subjected to changes we did not initiate, both doctor and patient feel as if they are churning out-of-control in the gigantic Cuisinart of the system. Doctors because they've gone from being independent entrepreneurs to being employees who must obey rules and regulations. Patients because they may have been enrolled instead of enrolling, and may also have to abide by rules and regulations. But there is no one who is going to represent your individual needs as well as you.

Up until now, the corporations that own HMOs have been so business-minded they haven't been listening enough to either side—patients' or doctors'. Since health care has become an industry, it seems it has become a matter of dollars and cents. And those in leadership positions know more about running a profitable business than they do about providing excellent health care. But remember that in the traditional fee-for-service days, practice was a matter of dollars and cents.

Even now, although it seems that nobody cares, everyone in the system basically is accountable to you. It's up to us, as patients, to be aware and try to have an impact. You are the customer, you are the consumer, and the services are designed for you. Besides finding your way in the system, you face the continuing challenge of navigating your own encounters with the physician. If anything, this applies more so now that both you and your physician are under more stress and must adapt to changes—changes that often feel more like losses. All the guiding principles that have been basic to getting the most out of your relationship with the doctor still prevail.

Inform yourself about his or her practice. Find out how to reach your doctors during the day, night, and weekend. Don't wait too long to call either for appointments or for urgent care. Prioritize your concerns. Plan for your visit. Develop realistic expectations. Work on your skills for formulating and expressing your concerns and articulating your expectations. Be trusting, but don't expect magic. Do not fear asking questions and insist on clear explanations. Take joint responsibility with the physician for decisions about your own health care. Expect empathy, but not pity. You expect the doctor to explore your views, so try to look at your situation from the doctor's perspective. Respect his or her professional expertise as a physician, but not at the expense of your own self-awareness or common sense.

For us doctors, the new system presents different challenges and we are also having to make adaptations. Lots of interns and medical students ask me, *"Would you go into medicine again if things were the way they are now when you started?"* My answer continues to be *"Yes!"* Most other doctors feel the same way. We've all heard HMO war stories, but remember that patients have been complaining about doctors and medical practice throughout history. Patients used to complain about their doctors, now they are complaining about the system.

The basic, crucial relationship—the interaction between doctor and patient—is the same in all the different systems. Doctors still need to find out what's wrong and help you. Patients' needs basically have not changed. And so it's up to both doctors and patients to adapt to the new system and preserve the central, helping relationship. Remember, it is the quality of the relationship between doctor and patient that predicts good health care, not the amount of time you spend with the doctor.

NOTES

▼
▼

So, What Did the Doctor Say?

1. Personal communication.
2. H. B. Beckman and R. M. Frankel. "The effect of physician behavior on the collection of data." *Annals of Internal Medicine 101:* 692–696, 1984.
3. S. Greenfield, S. Kaplan, and J. E. Ware. "Expanding patient involvement in care: Effects on patient outcomes." *Annals of Internal Medicine 102:* 520–528, 1985.

What Went Wrong?

1. American Academy of Pediatrics, policy statement. "The Dorman-Delcato treatment of neurologically handicapped children." *Pediatrics* 70:810–812, 1982.
2. B. M. Korsch and V. F. Negrete. "Doctor-patient communication." *Scientific American 227:* 66–74, 1972.

Why Don't I Follow My Doctor's Advice?

1. D. Meichenbaum and D. C. Turk. *Facilitating Treatment Adherence: A Practitioner's Guidebook.* New York: Plenum, 1987.
2. L. W. Buckalew and R. E. Sallis. "Patient compliance and medication perception." *Journal of Clinical Psychiatry 42:* 49–53, 1986.

3. B. M. Korsch, E. K. Gozzi, and V. Francis. "Gaps in doctor-patient communication." *Pediatrics 42:* 855–871, 1968; V. Francis, B. M. Korsch, and M. J. Morris. "Gaps in doctor-patient communication." *New England Journal of Medicine 280:* 535–540, 1969; and Korsch and Negrete. *Op. cit.,* 66–74.

4. L. S. Neinstein, D. Stewart, and N. Gordon. "Effect of physician dress style on patient-physician relationship." *Journal of Adolescent Health Care 6:* 456–459, 1985.

5. H. Leventhal. "Findings and theory in the study of fear communications." *Advances in Experimental Psychology 5:* 119–157, 1970.

6. S. H. Kaplan, S. Greenfield, and J. E. Ware. "Assessing the effects of physician-patient interactions on the outcomes of chronic disease." *Medical Care. 27:* S110–S127, 1989.

Where Is the Truth?

1. Hippocrates. "Decorum" in *Hippocrates* with an English translation by W. H. S. Jones. New York: G.P. Putnam's Sons, 1923.

2. O. W. Holmes. *Medical Essays.* Boston: Houghton Mifflin, 1911.

3. E. Cassell. *Talking with Patients, Vol. 1: The Theory of Doctor-Patient Communication.* Cambridge: MIT Press, 1985.

4. D. Spiegel. "Effect of psychosocial treatment on survival of patients with metastatic breast cancer." *Lancet 2* (8668): 888–891, 1989.

5. Personal communication.

6. R. B. Deber, N. Kraetschmer, and J. Irvine. "What role do patients wish to play in treatment decision making?" *Archives of Internal Medicine 156:* 1414–1420, 1996.

7. C. Lerman, S. Narod, et al. "BRCA1 testing in families with hereditary breast-ovarian cancer." *Journal of the American Medical Association 275:* 1885–1892, June 26, 1996.

Does Your Doctor Seem Unfeeling?

1. J. T. Ptacek and T. L. Eberhardt. "Breaking bad news." *Journal of the American Medical Association 276,* No.6: 496–501, 1996.

How Do Doctors Get That Way?

1. R. E. Miller, J. V. Murphy, and I. A. Mirsky. "Relevance of facial expression and posture as cues in communication of affect between monkeys." *Archives of General Psychiatry 1*: 480–488, 1959.
2. E. R. Werner and B. M. Korsch. "The vulnerability of the medical student: Posthumous presentation of L. L. Stephens' ideas." *Pediatrics 57:* 321–328, 1976.

Do I Have to Go to the Doctor?

1. E. G. Jaco. "Definitions of health and illness in the light of American values and social structure," in *Patients, Physicians and Illness*. New York: Free Press, 1972.
2. M. Verres. "Touch me." *Journal of the American Medical Association 276*, No.16: 1285–1286, 1996.

When Your Child Is Sick

1. C. E. Lewis, M. A. Lewis, A. Lorimer, and B. B. Palmer. "Child-initiated care: The use of school nursing services by children in an "adult-free" system." *Pediatrics 60* (4): 499–507, October 1977.

The Hospital

1. D. L. Roter and J. A. Hall. *Doctors Talking with Patients/Patients Talking with Doctors*. Westport, Conn.: Auburn House, 1992.
2. Personal communication.

Getting the Most Out of Managed Care

1. N. Korsch. *Op. Cit.*, 66–74.

SELECTED READINGS

Balint, M. *The Doctor, His Patient and the Illness*. New York: International University Press, 1972.

Bloom, W. S. *The Doctor and His Patient: A Sociological Interpretation*. New York: Russell-Sage Foundation, 1963.

Cassell, E. *The Healer's Art*. New York: Penguin, 1979.

Duff, R. S., and Hollingshead, A. B. *Sickness and Society*. New York: Harper & Row, 1987.

Katz, J. *The Silent World of Doctor and Patient*. New York: Free Press, 1984.

Lipkin, M., Jr., Putnam, S. M., and Lazare, A., eds. *The Medical Interview*. New York: Springer-Verlag, 1995.

Roter, D. L., and Hall, Judith A. *Doctors Talking with Patients/Patients Talking with Doctors*. Westport, Conn.: Auburn House, 1992.

Stewart, M., and Roter, D., eds. *Communicating with Medical Patients*. Newbury Park: Sage Publications, 1989.

INDEX

▼
▼